Clean & Lean Diet

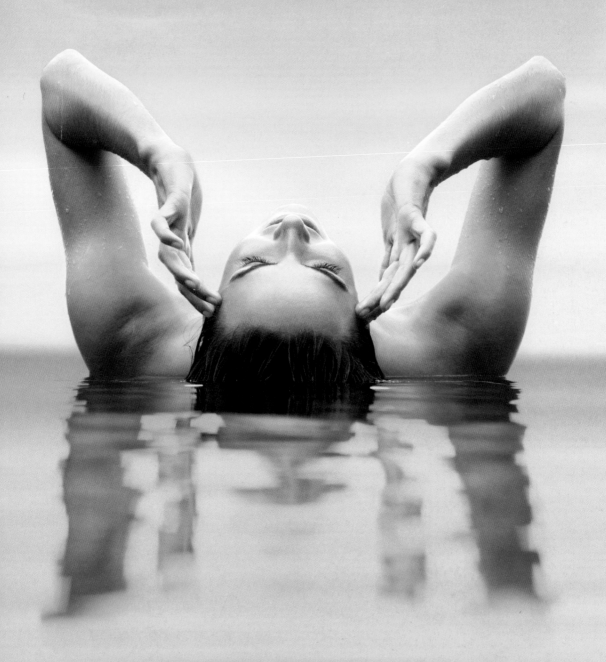

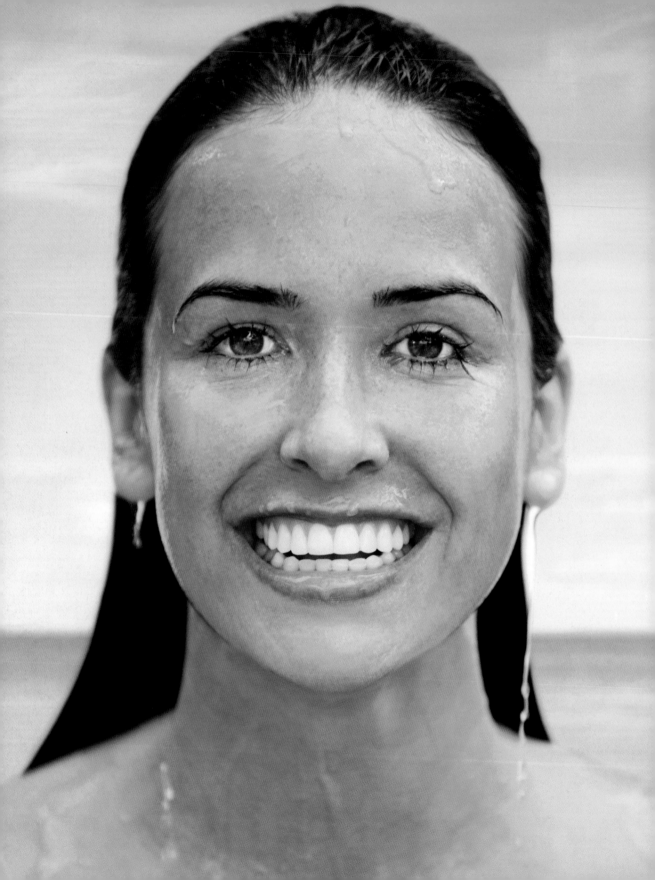

Clean & Lean Diet

14 days to your best-ever body

James Duigan, fitness expert for *The Times* (UK), and co-owner of Bodyism, London's premier fitness studio, is one of the world's top personal trainers. His many celebrity clients include Elle Macpherson, Rosie Huntington-Whiteley and Hugh Grant. James and his gym have been featured in *Vogue*, *InStyle*, *Glamour*, *Harpers Bazaar*, and *Marie Claire*.

James Duigan

with Maria Lally

Photography by Sebastian Roos and Will Heap
Shot on location at the One & Only Resort, Mauritius

KYLE BOOKS

First published in Great Britain in 2010 by
Kyle Books
An imprint of Kyle Cathie Ltd.
Distributed by National Book Network
(800) 462 6420
www.nbnbooks.com

ISBN 978-1-906868-38-3

Text © 2010 by James Duigan and Maria Lally
Recipes pages 78, 79, 81, 83–92, 102, 104, 106–09 © 2010 by
Nina Harris
Design © 2010 by Kyle Cathie Limited
Location and exercise photographs © 2010 by Sebastian Roos
Recipe photographs © 2010 by Will Heap

Editor Judith Hannam
Design Lisa Pettibone
Models Christiane McMillan, Natalie Bomgren
Location styling Emilie Lind
Recipe home economy and styling Polly Webb Wilson
Copy editor Anne Newman
Americanizer Stephanie Schwartz
Production Gemma John

Library of Congress Control Number: 2010934833

Printed and bound by Craft Print International Limited

The information and advice contained in this book are
intended as a general guide. Neither the author nor the
publishers can be held responsible for claims arising from the
inappropriate use of any remedy or exercise regime. Do not
attempt self-diagnosis or self-treatment for serious or long-
term conditions before consulting a medical professional or
qualified practitioner. Do not begin any exercise program or
undertake any self-treatment while taking other prescribed
drugs or receiving therapy without first seeking professional
guidance. Always seek medical advice if any symptoms persist.

Contents

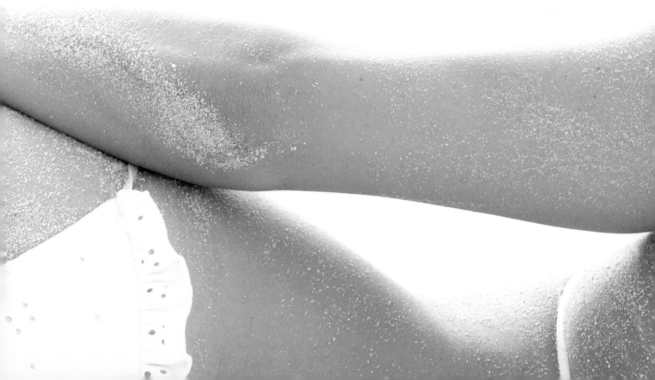

Foreword by Elle Macpherson

I met James in the mid-90s before I became pregnant with my first son. As I watched him train at the gym, where I was on the running machine, I was fascinated by his elegance and by his effortless exercising. He was lean and strong but not pumped up—he was focused and self-aware. I immediately wanted to work with him, as he seemed to have something I hadn't seen in other trainers.

We started working together and he immediately understood that I wanted to maintain a long, lean, healthy body while retaining my femininity and curves.

He also knew we didn't have the luxury of time or the headspace to be obsessive at the gym.

We worked on my body, attitude, diet, balance, strength, and consistency.

James' approach is non-gimmicky and straightforward. He works from the inside out—clearing the body and the mind and doing varied exercises.

Soon I became in the best shape ever—mentally and physically.

We've been through a lot together over the last ten years or so, including my second pregnancy, numerous photo shoots, and red carpet appearances. We're both Australian and we love an outdoor lifestyle.

A true testament to his workouts is that, ten years on, we still train together because he keeps it relevant and fun—it works! There is literally nobody better in the world than James for getting a woman's body into amazing shape.

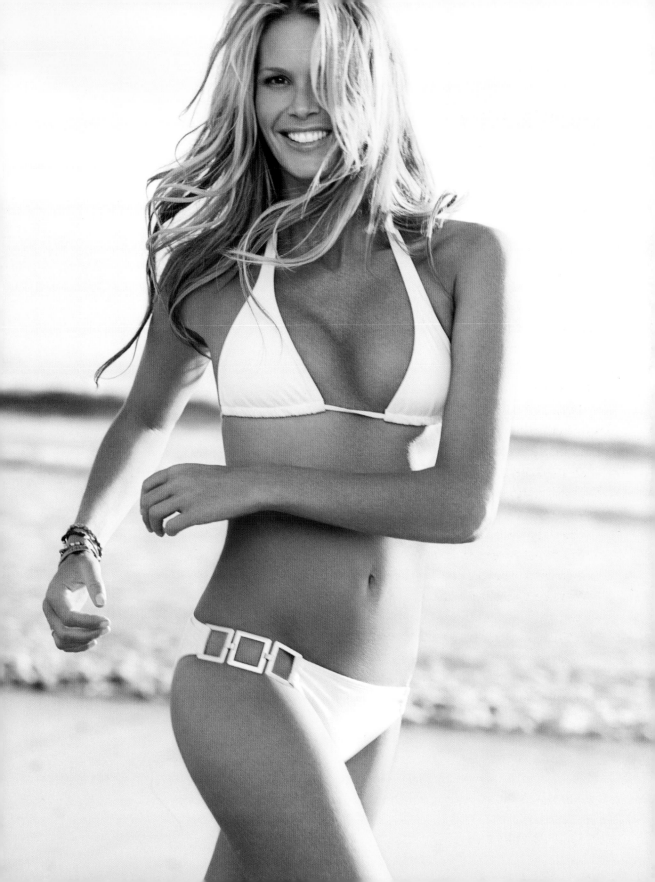

Introduction by James Duigan

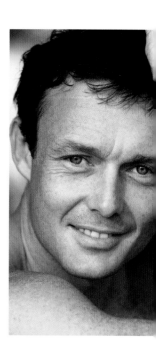

Let's get one thing straight: your body really, really wants to be slim. It wants to be lean and light, and strong and healthy, simply because that's the way it's designed to be—lean and healthy is its natural state.

Don't believe the myth that the human body clings on to fat. It doesn't—because it knows that's not the way it functions best. However, when you eat or drink processed foods, alcohol, bad fats, and refined sugar, your body becomes overloaded with toxins. It's these toxins, and not your body, that cling on to the fat. And because of this, you end up with squidgy bits of flesh around the thighs and hips and on your back, plus rolls of padding around the waist, as well as a distended tummy that becomes more bloated through-out the day.

But if your body looked the way it should—lean and light—you'd feel pretty amazing. You wouldn't need coffee or a muffin packed with sugar to help you function in the morning, despite the fact that you've just had seven or eight hours' sleep. You wouldn't get that crashing tiredness in the afternoon that only more coffee or a chocolate cookie can (briefly) keep at bay. And you wouldn't have that insatiable desire for something sweet after lunch and dinner, or any time in between.

Instead, you'd wake up after a good night's sleep, feeling energized and refreshed. Your energy levels would be high, as would your concentration levels, sex drive, and mood.

So your job now is to make the decision to take action and stick to it. And I'm going to show you how to do it: how to eat, how to exercise, and how to ensure that you stay motivated.

First off, it's important to understand that your weight and health are not separate issues. Being overweight is a symptom of being unhealthy. Focus on your health and the weight will drop off. You will also need to learn the difference between an excuse and a reason. Be brutally honest: if you really want something, you'll find a way to get it. So if you find yourself saying, "I didn't have time to exercise today" or, "I didn't have time to prepare healthy food," let me ask you this: would you have found time if your life depended on it? Well, it does.

You must believe you can do this. It doesn't matter how often you have failed in the past—your past does not equal your future. What matters now is focusing on what you want, identifying what you need to get it, and taking consistent action. Your health and happiness are important, so stand strong.

Create a support system for yourself. Explain to those around you what you are trying to do and how much it means to you. Ask your friends and family for help; if they choose not to encourage you, they may not be the best people to be around right now. Making yourself accountable will also help: tell people you have cut out alcohol, bread, or whatever, and this will help you stick with it. Take it one step at a time, so that you don't get overwhelmed.

With the help of this book, you will soon find out just how easy it is to become clean and lean for life. And you won't need to exercise for hours every day, either; in fact, you'll learn that too much exercise can actually slow down your weight-loss efforts, and that all you really need to do is a few simple moves each day.

You don't have to follow every single rule religiously—it's better that you stick wholeheartedly to those you can manage and that make the most difference to your energy levels, waistline, and life. Just try to stick to as many as possible, and you'll be blown away by the results.

So now read on, follow each easy step, and watch your body transform. I promise you, this works!

Chapter 1
Why Clean Equals Lean

This chapter will reveal…

▸ Why dieting is a waste of time

▸ Why toxins make you fat

▸ How organic food can help to make you slim

"Clean & lean" is a term I came up with that describes the ultimate approach to achieving the perfect body. The word "clean" here means a body that can deal effectively with toxins—one that can deal with the few that sneak in (via a glass of wine or chocolate bar) and flush them out successfully. And "lean" means just that—lean and healthy. It doesn't mean a body that's gym-honed to within an inch of its life or one that is scarily skinny. It means a lovely-looking body that's just the right side of athletic… a good mix of curvy, slim, and healthy. But if you want your body to be lean, it *has* to be clean.

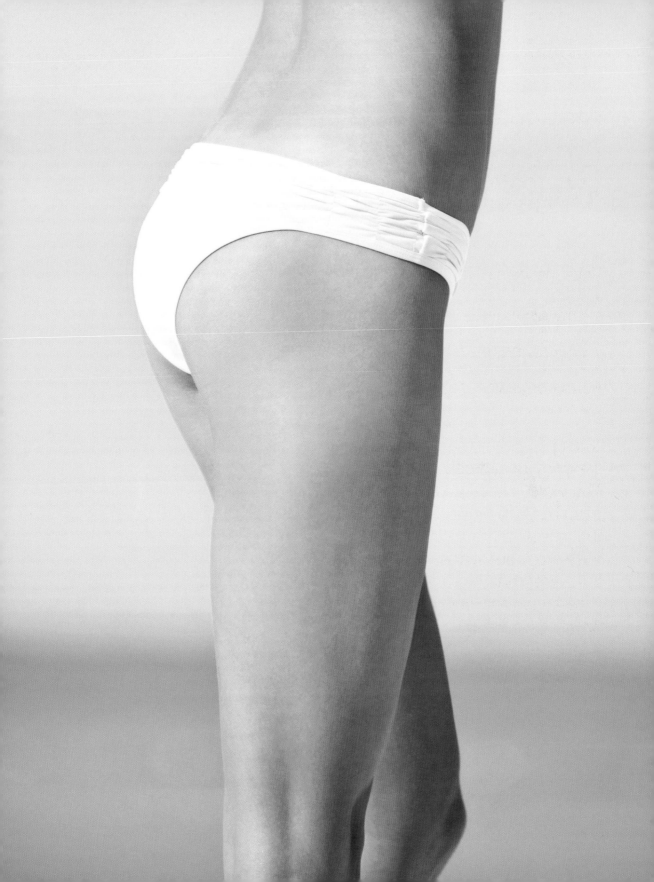

Why Dieting is a Waste of Time

I've spent years studying nutrition—and observing my clients—and I know this for certain. Sure, you can live on processed low-fat food and diet colas to lose weight. But your body will be so toxic that you'll find it hard to keep the weight off. I've seen this happen hundreds of times. People come to me who have been dieting for years—they tell me they've tried every single diet out there, yet they can't stay slim for long. They cut carbs, they count calories, they ban whole food groups, and they spend their lives weighing and measuring out food. But this type of dieting is a complete waste of time; it might help you to drop a dress size, but you'll gain it back again eventually because your body will still be toxic. And so the cycle of dieting, feeling miserable and deprived, losing and gaining weight continues.

My approach is different. There are no crazy rules, no measuring out food, no counting calories, and nothing is banned. You can have coffee every day—even during the 14-day Clean & Lean Kickstart. After this time, you can also have a blowout—an eat-whatever-you-like "cheat meal" (see p. 155) —once a week too. Yes, really! All you need to do is follow a few simple rules, which I'll explain in the course of this book, and get into a few easy habits that will become second nature after a while. You'll quickly and effortlessly become clean, then lean, as your body sheds the fat it's been holding onto for years. And it'll last a lifetime.

Why Toxins Make You Fat

Your body stores toxins (poisonous substances produced by living cells or organisms) in your fat cells. If you're dieting, your body will slowly lose fat, so the toxins will have nowhere to go but back into your system, making you feel tired, headachy, and generally unwell. This is why most people feel so rotten and tired within a few days of starting a diet. Your body then quickly decides it doesn't like feeling this way, so it holds onto fat in order to store the toxins (it's safer for toxins to be in fat cells, rather than floating around your body).

So if you're toxic, you're always going to find it hard to lose weight. Yes, you'll slowly drop pounds if you exercise enough and eat very little, but it'll be a long, hard process and one slip-up will see you a pound or two heavier

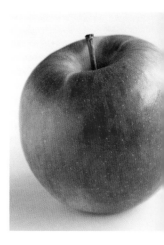

on the scales (your body will grab any chance it gets to cling onto fat). You'll also feel miserable, deprived, tired all the time, and you'll go to bed dreaming of chocolate bars every night. Then once you've lost weight, the real battle will begin as you try in vain to keep it off because the toxins will have turned your body into a fat-storing machine. Most people give up by this stage and just assume they're "meant" to be fat—that their body is just "designed that way."

And the harder the fat, the more toxic it is, and the more difficult it is to remove. When I see middle-aged men with solid, hard beer bellies it fills me with fear—the fat they're carrying around their stomachs is seriously toxic. Squidgy, soft fat is better; it's not great, but it's better than the really toxic hard stuff. As a general rule, the softer your fat bits are, the easier it will be to remove them. Hard fat also causes some serious health problems, like increased risk of diabetes, heart disease, and cancer, and while softer fat also increases your risk, the risk is smaller.

Lots of the very overweight people I see are actually also malnourished. Although we tend to associate malnourishment with skinniness, some of the most overweight people I've met are also the most malnourished. A toxic body doesn't digest or retain nutrients properly. And a high-calorie diet may not be high in vitamins and minerals. That's why fat people are so hungry—they're hungry for nutrients. A well-nourished body doesn't feel hungry: if you thoroughly chew a clean, lean meal (for example, a chicken salad full of all kinds of vegetables), you won't feel hungry afterward; but if you hurriedly eat a greasy burger and fries or a packaged meal, you'll feel hungry for something sweet afterward. That's because your body is left crying out for nutrients. Clean and lean food fills you up in a way that toxic food never can, plus chewing your food properly helps you stay nourished (and therefore less hungry) for longer because it releases the nutrients from your food.

So put simply: it's toxins that are stopping you from having the body you've always dreamed of. Clean them out of your system and you'll find losing weight is simple. To become truly clean, you need to clear out your excretory system, which is responsible for removing toxic waste from your body. So if you want a lean, lovely body, you need this system to be clean and functioning as best it can. The excretory system is made up of the three main detoxers—your skin (through sweating), your liver, and your kidneys.

I've cleaned out people's diets in the past, and the weight loss has been dramatic. And we're not even talking about crash diets or starvation here. These people were eating three meals a day, plus coffee and snacks, and they still dropped the weight effortlessly and quickly. How did they do it? They stopped eating and drinking toxins and they got clean.

Where are toxins found?

These are the most fattening toxins:

- Sugar
- Alcohol
- Soft drinks
- Processed foods
- Processed "diet" foods
- Excess caffeine
- Cortisol—the stress hormone

What makes foods clean?

Clean foods are those that:

- haven't changed much from their natural state—for example, an apple in a bowl still resembles the apple on the tree, whereas a potato chip (having been heavily processed) looks nothing like a potato
- don't need any added fake flavor
- don't last for months and months; they spoil in the fridge or cupboard
- contain fewer than five or six ingredients
- have no ingredients that you can't pronounce or recognize
- don't list sugar as their main ingredient (or as one of the first three)
- don't make you feel bloated, gassy, or uncomfortably full
- satisfy you, so that you're not hungry after eating them.

Top tip!

▶ If it couldn't swim, fly, or run, or it didn't grow off the land—don't eat it!

What else makes you toxic?

Anybody who doesn't live on a beautiful, deserted tropical island—so most of us—will come into daily contact with toxins. Fumes from cars, dirt in the air, medication, toxins in cleaning products, tap water—you name it, it's toxic. But let's face it, we'd lead a pretty miserable (not to mention weird) life if we tried to avoid these thing altogether. Several people also argue that our bodies are perfectly capable of dealing with toxins—and they're right, up to a point, because our bodies are designed to cope with them. Unfortunately, however, we're exposed to so many of them nowadays—especially in food and drink— that we've become overloaded. So it makes sense to limit our bodies' exposure toxins in the first place. We can do this by keeping our food as clean and lean as possible and by limiting our exposure to toxins from other sources. Don't forget—fewer toxins equals a leaner body.

Tap water, in my opinion, is fairly toxic and best avoided. A 2008 inquiry by the Associated Press found traces of prescription and over-the-counter medication in drinking water supplies across the USA. These traces were incredibly small, so there's no need to panic, but it makes sense to make sure that everything you eat and drink is as clean as possible, so buy a water filter jug and keep it in your fridge. You can also get a filter attached to your faucet at home, but this will be more expensive.

Antioxidants

I'll be talking about antioxidants a lot in this book. Antioxidants are substances that protect your cells from the harmful effects of free radicals (found in the environment, chemicals, rays from the sun, and tobacco smoke). These free radicals damage your cells and basically age you—from your skin to your heart. Antioxidants mop up free radicals and slow down the aging (and therefore degenerative) process. They are mostly found in brightly colored fruits and vegetables, especially those with high levels of vitamin A, C, and E and lycopene.

Antioxidant-rich foods include:
▶ tomatoes (they're packed with lycopene)
▶ dark red, blue, or black fruits with thin skin (blueberries, blackberries, strawberries, raspberries)
▶ sweet potatoes
▶ red, green, yellow, and orange peppers
▶ avocados
▶ dark greens (spinach, arugula, etc.)
▶ Bodyism Super Green and Red powders— Super Green is packed full of natural antioxidants derived from organic vegetables, while Super Reds are from organic fruits.

Are some toxins worse than others?

Absolutely. For example, caffeine is better for us than alcohol. In moderation and when drunk properly (see Chapter 3 for more information on this), coffee can actually burn fat, give you a great hit of antioxidants, and improve your performance in the gym. It's only when you have too much of it that it becomes fattening because it places stress on the adrenal glands, disturbs sleep, dehydrates you, and may stop you drinking enough water. However, one cup of coffee a day is a good thing if you drink good-quality, ideally organic, black coffee with a splash of organic milk.

Alcohol, on the other hand, has few if any benefits. There is some evidence that red wine is an antioxidant but otherwise alcohol is toxic and causes damage to almost every part of the body, from the internal organs to the skin and the waistline.

After 14 days, can I reintroduce toxins?

By the time you've read this book, I promise that you won't view foods like cake and chocolate in the same way. I appreciate you may still want them occasionally, and the Clean & Lean plan allows for that. Throughout the book, you'll get to meet my clients, many of whom need to take their own clients out for dinner or drinks, and who have a really sweet tooth and want chocolate! You'll find out how they've incorporated these things into their life while staying clean and lean.

So to answer the question: during the 14-day Clean & Lean Kickstart, you can have a cup of (organic) tea or coffee every day. After this, you can have up to two cups a day. You're not allowed any alcohol during the 14-day kickstart and, ideally, I'd like you to avoid it for a further four weeks after that. However, if you absolutely must have it, only drink once a week for four weeks and then have only red wine or clear spirits (go for Grey Goose vodka—it's the least processed one). After that, you can drink in moderation (I'll explain how to make healthy choices in Chapter 3). Cutting back on alcohol will give you such speedy weight loss that I promise you it will be worth it. My slimmest clients don't really drink (Elle included), because they see a bottle of wine for what it is—a bottle full of sugar and toxins that makes you fat: large amounts enlarge your liver so that your body doesn't metabolize fat as well; it's full of sugar, which you store as fat around your waist; and it increases your hunger (when you're drinking it and the next day), which weakens your willpower.

Why Organic Food Helps You Slim

Organic food is likely to contain fewer toxins (such as pesticides) and other additives found in nonorganic food (such as aspartame, tartrazine, MSG, and hydrogenated fats). Farming methods today are very often driven by profit: pesticides are sprayed onto crops to keep the produce alive for as long as possible (for example, the longer a strawberry stays fresh, the more it's likely to sell, keeping profits higher for the farmers and the food manufacturers). Similarly, nonorganic animals are fed more cheaply (and with more toxins) than organic ones.

Organic foods also contain more health-boosting minerals and vitamins, higher levels of vitamin C, calcium, magnesium, iron, antioxidants, and omega 3 fatty acids—all of which can help to make you healthier, stronger and slimmer. Take organic milk, for example, which- contains up to 68 per cent more omega 3 essential fatty acids than regular milk, helping your body to burn fat around your waist (more on this in Chapter 5).

Genetically modified (GM) crops and ingredients are banned under organic standards. However, GM crops are also fed to non-organic livestock, which ends up as nonorganic pork, bacon, milk, cheese, and other dairy products found in our supermarkets. So always, always pick organic food, wherever possible—especially when it comes to meat, dairy, and eggs.

To give you a clearer picture, here's my "Bad, Better and Best" guide to buying organic:

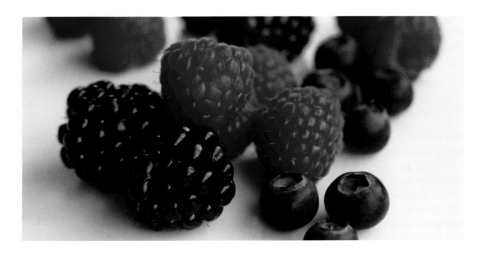

Bad	Better	Best
Chicken breasts	Free-range chicken breasts	Organic chicken breasts
Supermarket eggs	Free-range eggs	Organic eggs
Margarine	Butter	Organic butter
Instant coffee (coffee is one of the most sprayed plants in the world, plus processing it into an "instant" form further depletes nutrients.	Espresso (less processed than instant coffee); no milk, sugar or other additives	Organic espresso with organic cream – pesticide and herbicide-free (the cream slows the digestion of the caffeine)
Strawberry yogurt (remember, all the overripe fruit is put into yogurt, meaning more sugar and fewer nutrients)	Strawberries (500 lbs of pesticide per acre is sprayed on nonorganic strawberries—yuck!)	Organic strawberries (remember— the thinner the skin, the more pesticides are absorbed into the fruit; this is why you should always choose organic for berries and cherries)
Supermarket steaks (supermarkets buy cheaply in bulk and often from overseas, which means a longer time from the farm to your table)	Steaks bought from a butcher (these steaks are usually from locally reared animals)	Organic steaks (free from hormones, antibiotics, and nitrates)
Cow's milk	Goat's milk	Organic rice milk or oat milk
Iceberg lettuce (basically green water with almost no nutrients; the lettuce of today has one-twentieth of the nutrients it had fifty years ago, due to severely mineral-depleted soil)	Spinach (very high in magnesium, calcium, antioxidants, and chloro-phyll, which cleanses your blood and helps detox your liver)	Organic spinach (as with nonorganic, but with lots more nutrients)
Dried fruit	Fresh fruit	Organic fruit
Waxed apples (the really shiny apples you see at the supermarket are coated in wax; they look better, but the wax actually drags nutri-ents from them)	Loose apples in a bag	Organic apples (they may not look as pretty, but they don't contain any nasty toxins, either)
Dried apricots (high in sugar and sulfates that destroy vitamins in the foods they preserve)	Fresh apricots	Organic apricots
White rice (in some countries the rice fields have been sprayed with so much pesticide that the ground water has become contaminated)	Brown rice (this still has the brown skin on it, increasing the fiber content)	Organic brown rice (lots of fiber and no pesticides)

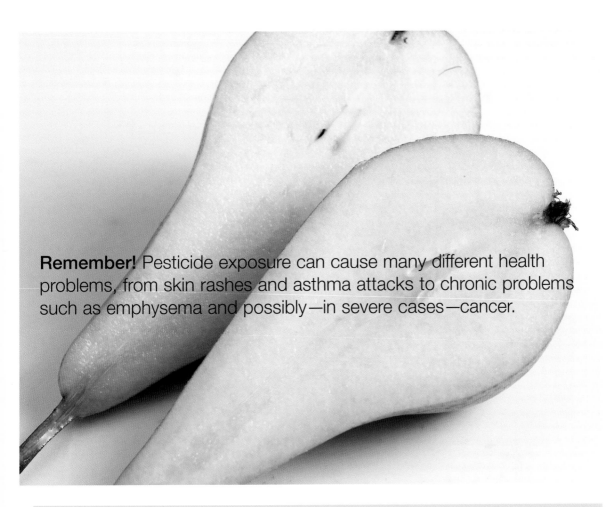

Remember! Pesticide exposure can cause many different health problems, from skin rashes and asthma attacks to chronic problems such as emphysema and possibly—in severe cases—cancer.

KATE'S STORY

Thirty-year-old Kate walked through my door on a mission. She was getting married four months later and wanted to drop three dress sizes—and it was either me or plastic surgery that was going to help her do it. She was willing to listen and take on board whatever I said; she looked me right in the eye and said that nothing on earth would make her stray from what I told her to do.

I put her on a hardcore version of the Clean & Lean plan for two weeks, during which she ate nothing but fish and green vegetables for breakfast, lunch, and dinner. She also had a Super-skinny Fat-burning Bodyism drink every day (see p. 158).

Within two weeks, Kate had dropped a dress size and was glowing. Within two months, she'd got to a size six (her goal) without any help from the scalpel and without starving herself either. Brides are the best people to train because there are few human beings on the planet more motivated to strip fat!

Chapter 2
Why Sugar Is Not So Sweet

This chapter will reveal…

▸ Why sugar is addictive

▸ Why sugar is so bad for you

▸ How to give sugar up

Most of us love sugar—I know I do. And with 128 million tons of it produced worldwide each year, it seems I'm not the only one with a sweet tooth. So why do we love it so much?

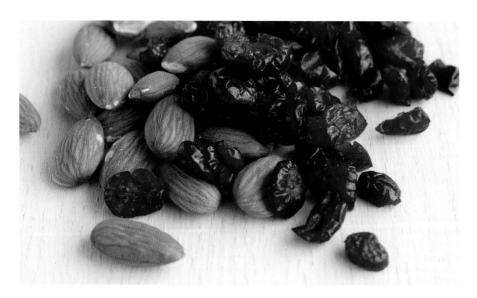

Why Sugar is Addictive

Sugar is perfectly designed to hook us in. It comes to us in the form of pretty pink icing, fluffy marshmallows, gorgeous-looking cupcakes, light cakes with jam in the middle, and creamy chocolate. In fact, just about everything sugary looks and smells delicious.

I was watching my baby cousin at his first birthday party the other day, when he got his first hit of sugar from his birthday cake. You could see his little face light up; he loved that sugar and he just wanted more. It was almost scary.

But, in reality, there's nothing to love about refined sugar. It makes us put on weight, increases the size of our liver, makes us unwell, and ages us inside and out, leaving us tired, fat, and wrinkled. As well as being highly addictive, refined sugar drags valuable nutrients out of our body, and it's the number one reason why, for the first time in history, the children of this generation are predicted to die younger than their parents because they're going to end up fatter and sicker. This is happening because sugar is a big business with a massive marketing campaign behind it, so it's able to target us from a very early age, making addicts of us all.

Why sugar is physically addictive

Sugar has a similar effect on the brain to painkilling drugs like morphine and other opiates (such as heroin). These types of drugs produce an almost instant feeling of pleasure, calm, and satisfaction, making them incredibly addictive. When the food manufacturers figured this out, they began producing foods full of sugar. Back in the 1950s, sugar would mainly be found in homemade cakes, but now it's pumped into almost all processed foods, alcoholic and soft drinks, and even so-called "healthy" foods (such as breakfast cereals) and foods aimed at children. As a result, we're all more addicted and fatter than ever.

Many of us turn to something sugary for "energy"—and technically, it is a form of energy. But it's a bad type. So yes, you will get a quick burst after eating a chocolate bar, but about ten minutes after that you'll feel even more tired than you were before. That's because sugar quickly hits the bloodstream, creating a rapid rise in blood sugar (a "spike"). But, just as quickly, you then crash (due to insulin being produced from the pancreas), leaving you exhausted. A far better way of getting energy is to eat complex carbohydrates (low-GI fruits, berries), clean and lean proteins, vegetables, drink plenty of water, and exercise regularly. If you do all these things, you won't need to rely on something as toxic as sugar to keep you energized.

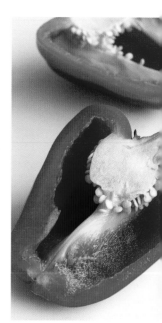

Studies also suggest that the ability to tell between sweet and bitter is hard-wired into our DNA. It helped us to survive in cavemen times when we needed to know the difference between what was poisonous and what was safe to eat. We are also one of the only animals that cannot produce our own vitamin C—we need to get it from what we consume. And vitamin C is found mostly in things that are sweet. So it's reasonable to assume that we're hard-wired to want food that is sweet and probably abundant in vitamin C (most vitamin-C rich fruits like berries and oranges are very sweet). This wasn't so much of a problem in the days when we had to hunt and gather our own food—there were no junk-filled, sugary treats on offer back then. These days, however, they're everywhere and sugar is far more available and comes in far worse forms. After all, the natural sugar found in fruit is one thing but the processed rubbish found in sweets and cakes is something else altogether.

Why sugar is emotionally addictive

For most of us, when we were growing up, sugary foods were used as a "reward" by our parents, grandparents, and almost everybody else we knew as children. If we got good grades at school, we'd be given candy on the way home, to say, "Well done." When we stayed with our grandparents and behaved ourselves, we got cake (actually I got cake at my grandparents' house, no matter what I did; I think it was their way of thanking my dad for being such a cheeky teenager—they'd send me home teetering on the brink of a sugar-induced tantrum). When we felt sad because we'd scraped our knee, we were given cookies to cheer us up. And as for birthdays—we'd get a huge cake, literally drenched in sugar, to celebrate. So is it any wonder that by the time we reached our teens, we'd learned to associate sugary foods with happy times and making ourselves feel better?

I had a client once who was hopelessly addicted to sugar. When she first came to see me, her diet was appalling. She had to eat something sugary every day, especially after meals or whenever she was stressed or sad. When

I dug a little deeper, it turned out that her mother was seriously ill when she was very young, and her father had to take care of her a lot when her mother was in and out of hospital. As a toddler, if she was upset or had trouble sleeping, her father would dip her pacifier in some honey to soothe her. As a result, she always turned to sugar for comfort.

Many of us do exactly the same thing as this client: when we're heart-broken, lonely, sad, or stressed, we turn to sugar to make us feel better, gorging on ice cream, cake or chocolate to cheer ourselves up. But guess what? Sugary foods don't cheer us up. They make us fat, stressed, old-looking, and ill. So the next time you go to eat something sugary because you've been dumped or you've had a bad day at work, stop and ask yourself: "Will this make my problems better or worse?" Look past the pretty pink icing and see sugar for the fattening toxin that it is.

Why Sugar is so Bad for You

Over the last fifty years, the Western world has doubled its consumption of processed sugar (the type found in cookies, soft drinks, and ice cream, for example) and, during this time, rates of obesity and heart disease have soared. Of course, sugar isn't solely responsible—but it is largely to blame. If you think I'm being overly dramatic about it, Google "Harmful effects of processed sugar" and you'll get about six million links. Millions of people (especially in the USA and the UK, where processed sugar consumption is highest) are fat, unwell, and living uncomfortably, getting by on all sorts of medications just to keep their overloaded bodies going.

MARIE'S STORY

"I used to be a huge sugar addict. I saw a chocolate bar in the afternoon as a break from work. I also loved a cupcake or a muffin with my latte and some biscuits with a hot cup of tea. But James made me realize that it wasn't the sugar I was enjoying, but the things I associated it with. In fact, when I thought about it, I felt worse after eating it. It made my stomach bloat and my energy levels plummet. When I stopped eating it, I felt lighter, slimmer, and my skin glowed. Now I rarely touch the stuff, and I don't miss it at all."

In the autumn of 2009, the American Heart Association (AHA) released a statement urging people to cut back on processed sugar. They advised that women should have no more than six teaspoons a day, which is around 100 calories' worth (and remember, this is the absolute most you should be having – ideally you shouldn't really have any at all, unless it comes from natural sources like fruit), yet the average American has 22 teaspoons a day! To give you an idea, just one can of diet drink contains around eight teaspoons of sugar; imagine how much sugar you're eating if you add biscuits, cakes, sweets and everything else sugary on top of that.

Several studies have tried to bring people's attention to the effects of eating too much sugar on everything from their waistlines to their mood. Yes, that's right – too much sugar can actually make you depressed. Is that cupcake still really so tempting now?

What eating sugar can do to you

Sugar makes you fat: your body cannot process too much of it, so it gets stored as fat. Plus it also makes fat-burning even harder – if you're eating sugar every day, all the gym sessions in the world won't shift that excess flab.

As we've seen (see p. 21), sugar is also addictive, so once you start eating it, it's very hard to stop. This is why you very rarely find a packet of half-finished biscuits. Stop the cycle by not starting it.

Sugar leaches your body of vitamin B: any mental, physical or emotional stress drains vitamin B from your body – as does sugar – which causes exhaustion. If you add sugar on to the end of a stressed-out day, you're getting a double whammy of vitamin B depletion.

Burning body fat is all about controlling your insulin levels. But sugar spikes raise your insulin levels, leading to faster fat storage and this is the real reason why so many of us in the Western world are either overweight or obese. Sugar, not fat, is making us fatter. In a healthy, slim person, 40 per cent of the sugar they eat is converted straight to fat; in an overweight person, up to 60 per cent is converted straight to fat and stored right around their hips, stomach and thighs. Think about it: up to 60 per cent of that cupcake is heading straight for your tummy, hips and thighs, where it will remain for a very long time.

Sugar lowers energy levels: processed sugar causes a huge and damaging increase in your blood-sugar levels, giving you a quick burst of energy,

Top tips!

▶ Avoid overripe fruits. The riper a fruit is the more sugar it contains, meaning the higher your chance of storing that sugar as fat. So the next time you're choosing which piece of fruit to eat, don't go for the softest because it contains the most sugar.
▶ When eating an apple make sure you eat the skin, as this is where all the fibre is.
▶ The darker the fruit, the better. Dark fruits tend to have very thin skin, so they need to produce more antioxidants to protect themselves from the sun.

which is soon followed by a long, hard crash, leaving you tired, hungry and, eventually, fat.

Sugar wears out your organs: it forces your internal organs to cope with changes in your body chemistry which means that your kidneys and pancreas can become worn out long before you stop needing them. Hence the increase in late onset diabetes.

Too much sugar depletes stored-up vitamins and minerals in the body, which may impact on the immune system. So you become ill more frequently and for longer.

The worst offenders

White refined sugar—the stuff you get in envelopes and stir into your tea or cake mixtures.

Fruit juices—most commercial fruit juice is basically sugared water with all the fiber extracted and very little vitamin and mineral content. Within two minutes of squeezing fruit, most of the vitamins and minerals have been lost. It is best either to have a small glass of freshly squeezed juice or, better still, a piece of whole fruit.

Bad carbs —white, non-organic pasta, bread and rice, cereals and cereal bars are the worst offenders. Even seemingly healthy brown carbs (like whole wheat bread) contain sugar.

Alcohol—it's literally all sugar.

Cakes, sweets, cookies, ice cream—need I say more?

So-called "low-fat foods"—such as diet yogurts, most breakfast cereals (more on these in Chapter 3), health bars, muffins, and energy drinks, are all packed with sugar to give them flavor. A common trick of the food manufacturer is to label a food as being "low fat" when there was no fat in there to begin with. This is most common with breakfast cereals (again, see more on why you should never eat these in Chapter 3).

Any ingredient ending in "ose"—sugar is often hidden in words ending with "ose" (sucrose, maltose, lactose, dextrose, and fructose, for example). Another common name is "syrup," the very worst being "high-fructose corn syrup" (HFCS)—one of the cheapest sweeteners around, it boosts fat-storing hormones, while a recent study at the University of Pennsylvania found that it also increases the hunger hormone; it's found in candy, cereal bars, fruit drinks, ketchup, mayonnaise, pasta sauce, and even salad dressing, so always read the labels.

Anything that lists sugar—in any of its guises—in the first three ingredients.

You basically need to steer clear of any sweeteners, especially the artificial ones that are made of toxic chemicals. Remember that most packaged foods contain sweeteners along with other additives that you really want to avoid if you want a slim waist. Learn to read labels and avoid anything fake or toxic looking.

As a rough guide, here are some of the things you should be looking out for:

- High-fructose corn syrup
- White sugar
- Brown sugar
- Cane syrup
- Sucrose
- Dextrose
- Fructose

- Sucanat
- Beet sugar
- Maltose
- Sorbitol
- Mannitol
- Erythritol
- Aspartame
- Saccharin

- Nutrisweet
- Splenda
- Cyclamate
- Sucralose
- Acesulfame-K

How to Give Sugar Up

You really need to give sugar up if you want to be clean and lean. All the other things we're going to talk about in this book—like coffee—can be reintroduced once you've completed the 14-day Clean & Lean Kickstart. But sugar? It's so nasty, so toxic, and so utterly bad for you that it's better to just ditch it altogether. And here's how:

Don't use sugar as a reward

Ask yourself this—how is giving yourself early wrinkles, a bloated stomach, and fat around your middle a "reward"? See sugar for what it is— a nasty toxin that's dyed a pretty color to lure you in, and which then makes you fat and unwell. Reward yourself with something else instead, like a beauty treatment or a new book.

What about honey?

Raw honey, pure maple syrup, brown rice syrup, molasses (which are packed full of calcium, iron, B vitamins, and potassium), manuka honey (which is full of antioxidants), barley malt, stevia, and agave are all OK in moderation. But the key word here is "moderation." Like fruit, these things have their benefits—and they're certainly better for you than processed sugar—but they should still form only a small part of your diet.

If you are having a tough time quitting the habit and you need a little sweetness just to get through the day, I would recommend stevia. It's an herb that's 200 times sweeter than sugar. Another natural source of sweetness is xylitol, which you can buy in granulated form (so it's good for adding to hot drinks) and it releases energy slowly.

Eat plenty of chromium

Chromium helps to control your blood-sugar levels and banish sugar cravings. Good sources include eggs, molasses, liver, kidney, whole grains, nuts, mushrooms, and asparagus. It should not be eaten in large quantities if you are diabetic.

Supplement your diet with glutamine

Glutamine is an amino acid that squashes sugar cravings. It can be found in most health-food shops; take one tablespoon in a small glass of water whenever you get a sugar craving.

Include dark meat proteins in your diet

Sugar cravings often come from a lack of protein in your diet. Try eating darker meats, such as chicken legs, beef, and lamb. Dark meats contain more purines which have more satisfying nutrients than lighter meats, like chicken breasts or fish, so will help to prevent sugar cravings. In fact, if you're having a sugar craving, try having a slice of chicken or some nuts to banish the urge for sugar.

Take Bodyism supplements

Bodyism Body Brilliance supplements are packed with chromium plus cinnamon, which helps regulate your blood-sugar levels, boosting energy levels in turn and reducing sugar cravings throughout the day. Bodyism fish oil contains essential fatty acids, which are important for optimal health and can help reduce cravings for sugar, as your body is full of good fats.

Sugar in Fruit

The best form of sugar is raw fruit. So the next time you have a sweet craving, eat some in-season thin-skinned fruit, such as berries, apples, pears, cherries, or green grapes. Always make sure you eat these with protein and/or fat to slow down the speed at which the sugar hits your bloodstream.

Having said that, fruit—though packed with goodness—is still incredibly high in sugar, so don't eat too much of it. Yes, we all need "five a day" (i.e. five portions of fruit and vegetables a day), but the majority of this should come from vegetables. Go easy on fruit for a few weeks, and you'll be amazed at the difference it makes to your waistline, energy levels, and how much you bloat. Berries are the best fruit of all, so eat more of those than any other fruit.

How to eat sugar

If you feel you absolutely must have sugar, there are some rules you should stick to that will help with damage limitation:

Always eat sugar at the end of a meal (never before). By eating your protein first (remember—you must eat some protein with every meal), you leave less room for cravings, plus this prevents blood-sugar peaks and crashes.

Eat good sugar—as good as possible. That means raw, in-season, thin-skinned fruits (see above) or some really good-quality honey—though not too much. Once you start cutting back on sugar, you'll be amazed at how quickly you lose the taste for it, and when you do have some you'll need a lot less than you did before.

Never, ever eat sugar on its own (and this includes fruit and honey)— always eat with some protein and "good fat" (try a handful of nuts or a slice of meat or fish). This is because protein and fat slow the rate at which sugar floods into your bloodstream, and if sugar hits your bloodstream quickly— as it would after a huge cupcake, for example—you'll feel quickly high, then very quickly low. The slower it hits your blood, the less of a rush you'll get, which means less of a slump.

Here's my "Bad, Better and Best" guide on how to clean out bad, processed sugars from your diet and replace them with less toxic ones, once you've completed the 14-day Clean & Lean Kickstart (see Chapter 6). If you crave something in the "Bad" column, pick the one in the "Better" column instead. Or, for a body like Elle's, go for the one in the "Best" column!

Bad	Better	Best
White sugar	Brown sugar	Manuka honey
Chocolate-coated cookies	Piece of fruit	Fruit and nuts
Sweets	Dried fruit	Whole piece of fruit plus a handful of almonds
Breakfast cereal	Sugar- and wheat-free (oat–based) muesli	Super Breakfast (see p. 80 for the recipe)
Fruit-based cereal	Thick-skinned fruit salad—bananas, oranges, and watermelon	Thin-skinned fruit salad—cherries, blueberries, blackberries, straw-berries, and raspberries
Low-fat yogurt	Organic yogurt with fruit and honey	Raw organic yogurt with nuts
Ice pop	Fruit juice	Piece of fruit
Chocolate chip muesli bar	Nut bar—although held together with sugar, this has loads more protein than a muesli bar	A handful of raw nuts
Mars Bar	Cereal bar	A handful of raw nuts
Soft drink	Fruit juice	Water
Store-bought cake	Fresh cake from a bakery	Homemade cake, made with fruit as the sweetener and no white sugar
Cookies—full of salt, sugar, and bad fat	Oatcakes with nut butter	Rice cakes with turkey and avoca-do—the perfect blend of proteins, carbs, and good fats
Ice cream—milk held together with tons of sugar; most people can't digest dairy properly, which lowers your ability to burn fat	Natural organic yogurt with almonds—contains a lot less sugar and the protein helps fill you up	Fresh fruit—a small handful of berries and half an apple; these are rich in antioxidants to detox your system
Muesli/granola bar—stuck together with sugar; don't be fooled by their healthy image	Fresh fruit and nuts—contain fruit sugars and some complete protein bad fat	Raw vegetables—broccoli, celery, carrots, cucumber, and cauliflower are packed with nutrients and have very few calories
Chocolate bar—a convenient pocket-sized fat bomb	Fresh fruit and nuts	Raw vegetables with some avocado
Croissant—zero fiber and soaked in bad fats; probably the worst breakfast ever	Muffin from a health-food store	Raw vegetables with a little organic hummus—loads of fiber, vitamins, and minerals.

Chapter 3
Cut the CRAP*

*That's Caffeine, Refined Sugar, Alcohol, and Processed Foods

This chapter will reveal…

▸ Why too much coffee will make you fat

▸ Why alcohol should be avoided

▸ Why processed foods are so harmful

▸ Why you should avoid breakfast cereals

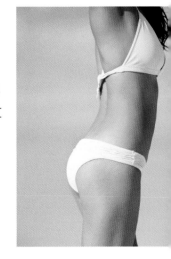

The four main toxins that cause our bodies to cling to fat are: **C**affeine, **R**efined sugar, **A**lcohol and **P**rocessed food. Or **CRAP**. There are plenty of other causes, which we'll discuss throughout the book, but these four are the big baddies, and when a client walks through my door, these are the ones I warn them about right away. We've looked at sugar already (the worst of all, which is why it got a chapter to itself), so I'm going to focus on the other three in detail here. But for a quick, so-easy-you-don't-even-need-to-think-about-it guide to staying slim, just think: I must avoid CRAP.

Why Too Much Coffee Will Make You Fat

Although caffeine is the first toxin I deal with here, it's actually the least fattening of the big four. In fact, I even allow you to have one cup of organic coffee (or tea) a day throughout the 14-day Clean & Lean Kickstart (see pages 68–73). This is because it is not so much caffeine itself that is so bad for you—it's the way that most of us drink it that's the problem. Excess caffeine (in the form of more than two cups of tea or coffee a day) stimulates your nervous system, causing your adrenals to pump out cortisol, a hormone that helps the body respond to stress. All that extra cortisol floats around your system for hours after you've drunk caffeine. So people who are drinking coffee or tea all day long are basically flooding their bodies with fat-storing hormones.

Then there are the calories that come from what I call "junk caffeine." That's coffee or tea with added sugar, or the iced coffees that come with flavored syrups or whipped cream. Caffeine past lunchtime also disrupts the way you sleep, and a lack of good-quality sleep encourages your body to store fat, especially around your middle. So drinking too much caffeine is literally like sticking an extra inch of flesh to your waistline. But you should avoid decaffeinated coffee too because the caffeine-removal process strips it of a lot of its goodness.

Having said all that, I love coffee just as much as the next person. But I use it to my advantage: on the plus side, caffeine can help the body burn fat and it also boosts your performance when you're exercising (have it at least half an hour beforehand). Organic coffee is also packed with antioxidants, and it's great for your digestion, helping to get your bowels going in the morning, keeping your body nice and clean and toxin-free. So go for one or two cups of organic coffee (or tea) a day, preferably in the morning. I love an Americano with a splash of full-fat organic milk or even cream; I also like a sprinkle of dried cinnamon on the top—it helps your body burn fat more efficiently and keeps blood-sugar levels steady. And the hit of flavor takes away the need for sugar and sweeteners.

Green tea also contains caffeine, but I love green tea and tell all my clients to drink it. It has less caffeine than coffee, so you can have more of it (up to six cups a day) and it also has more antioxidants. Plus it's a great detoxer for the body. It's especially good at getting rid of metal toxicity— that's basically toxins from the environment. Don't drink it right before bed though, as the caffeine will keep you awake. Instead, start drinking it first thing and stop at around 5 or 6 p.m. I tell my clients to brew a big pot of it, wait for it to cool down, then transfer it into a bottle and drink it cold throughout the day. It's up to you how you drink it, but limit yourself to six cups and make sure it's organic (it contains more antioxidants).

Opposite is my "Bad, Better and Best" guide to caffeine; always choose from the Best column if you can, or the Better column if you must. And unless you want a fat midsection, avoid the Bad column altogether.

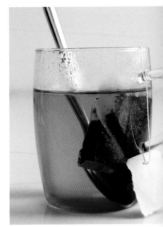

Why Alcohol Should Be Avoided

Alcohol is just about as bad as sugar, and the only reason why I've spent more time talking about sugar is because we're exposed to it all day long, whereas most of us are only likely to drink alcohol in the evenings.

Alcohol is basically a poison. For a start, it stimulates the production of estrogen in your bloodstream, which promotes fat storage (again, around your waist and tummy) and decreases muscle growth. If you have lots of lovely lean muscle, your body will burn calories all day long and you'll look lean, toned, and amazing. But drinking alcohol will decrease muscle mass, leaving you squidgy and out of shape. It's no coincidence that studies have shown that women's waist sizes have got bigger over the years, in line with the amount of alcohol they consume.

Alcohol is the simplest and most fattening sugar of all. That's why it's such a good carrier of medicine—it hits the bloodstream straight away. During the 14-day Clean & Lean Kickstart, I want you to give up alcohol completely. And if you can't manage two weeks without alcohol, then this isn't the book for you, I'm afraid. You really do have to cut it out for two whole weeks, after which you need to change the way you drink (more about this in Chapter 10).

Nearly all my clients like a drink. I train businessmen who go out with clients every night of the week and play soccer at the weekends, so I'm used to dealing with people whose life includes alcohol. I know it's hard to cut back on beer and white wine (two of the least clean drinks you can have) if

Bad	Better	Best
Instant coffee	Espresso	Espresso with organic cream
Black tea	Green tea	Caffeine-free herbal tea—peppermint, ginger, etc.
Milk chocolate (don't forget—chocolate contains caffeine)	Dark chocolate—more cocoa satisfies your chocolate craving sooner	Dark chocolate with nuts—added protein slows the digestion of the sugar, preventing an energy crash
Cola (any brand)	Caffeine-free energy drink—fewer artificial flavors and sugar	Fruit smoothie with seeds in it
High energy drinks	Guarana drink	Espresso with organic cream
Shop or café-bought iced coffee	Espresso blended with ice and milk	Espresso blended with ice and organic cream
Diet pills—these nearly all contain some form of caffeine	Green tea extract	Organic green tea
Instant hot drinks (tea, coffee, hot chocolate)—processed and full of junk	Espresso with heavy cream—the cream slows the effects of the caffeine	Caffeine free/herbal tea

your job involves wining and dining clients. But if you take in some of my changes, the results in your body will be amazing and it will be well worth it. So as a rule of thumb, I would recommend that you don't touch alcohol until you've reached your goal weight. Binge drinking at the weekend can take you two steps back, even after an otherwise healthy week; plus, a hangover makes you crave toxic foods.

Remember also that your liver is a fat-burning organ. So when it's busy trying to process a large glass of wine, it can't metabolize all the calories you've consumed during the day. That means for every drink you have, you're slowing down your metabolism, so your body isn't burning any fat. In fact, it's the reverse: it's storing it. Alcohol is like a fat bomb that explodes all over your body, especially over your stomach, waist, thighs, and backside.

Some of my clients say, "But surely red wine has some health benefits?" Well, the answer is yes and no—but mainly no. Red wine does contain a very small concentration of antioxidants (from the red grape skins, so pick red over white), but there are so few of these in a glass that it's hardly worth it. You'd have to drink so many bottles of red wine to get any benefits that the alcohol content would far outweigh the goodness anyway. If it's antioxidants you're after, you're far better off just grabbing a handful of red grapes (or any other food that's rich in antioxidants for that matter).

So alcohol, we've established, has few health benefits. It makes your body store fat, it stresses out your liver so it can't metabolize calories properly, and it will, eventually, make your face look old and wrinkled because of all the sugar it contains. However—and as a non-drinker it's hard for me to say this!—I realize that most of you will want to keep it in your life once you've completed the 14-day Kickstart. So here is my "Bad, Better and Best" guide to keeping alcohol consumption slightly healthier.

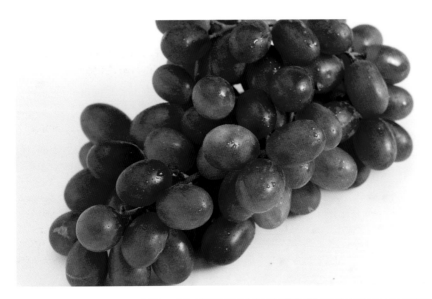

Beer Drinkers are Turning into Women!

Beer is one of the most sugary drinks there is, and when men drink too much of it their bodies become flooded with the female hormone estrogen. This results in fairly slim, undefined arms, a huge round belly, and "moobs" (man boobs). Many of my male clients arrive at my gym looking like this, and nothing makes them give up the booze faster than when I tell them, "All that beer is turning you into a woman!"

Bad	Better	Best
Beer—this is packed with sugar, yeast and alcohol and is the number-one fat-causing beverage in the world!	Organic beer—fewer pesticides and additives, meaning less stress on your liver (so a cleaner system); it's still loaded with calories though	Vodka, mineral water, and a squeeze of lemon or lime.
Wine—this is packed with sugar, yeast, and alcohol	Organic wine—see above	Gin and tonic with fresh lime—a clean, yeast-free spirit with minimal calories
Alcopop—packed with sugar and alcohol, these are designed to taste like soft drinks, so you drink yourself fat without noticing	Vodka and juice (from concentrate)—a lot less sugar than an alcopop	Vodka and freshly squeezed juice—alcohol with some nutritional value
White wine—packed with sugar, yeast, and alcohol	White wine spritzer—less sugar and less alcohol	Vodka and mineral water with fresh lemon or lime
Beer—see above	White wine—less sugar than beer	Red wine—has some antioxidant properties
Cocktails with cola mixers, such as Long Island Iced Tea—packed with sugar, fattening amounts of alcohol, plus caffeine	Cocktails with fruit mixers—fewer bad sugars and calories, so less of a fat bomb	Mocktails—nonalcoholic cocktails made with fresh juice
Vodka cocktails mixed with high energy drinks—equivalent to four coffees, plus a shot of alcohol; places your internal organs under stress	Vodka and lemon-lime soda	Vodka and mineral water with a squeeze of lemon or lime
Shots with a milky liqueur and dark spirit e.g. White Russian; packed with sugar, alcohol, and dairy—a sugary fat bomb	Single shot of clear spirit—one poison instead of several; also, less sugar	Shots are the beginning of the end! You really don't need them and your body will thank you for it in the morning if you just give them a pass
Malibu and cola—sugar with more sugar, plus caffeine and alcohol	Malibu and pineapple juice—some natural sugars, but still a fat bomb	Vodka with a fruit smoothie—clean spirit with plenty of nutrients and a little bit of fiber; sip it slowly and enjoy the taste

Remember! The more fresh flavors you put in your food, the better it will taste.

Why Processed Foods Are So Harmful

A processed food is one that's been altered from its natural state to make it cheaper, more convenient, or more attractive, or to extend its shelf life (or all four). All the foods you eat should be clean, meaning as close to their natural state as possible. But processed foods are far from that.

I hate processed foods. I mean, I really, really hate them. In my opinion they make you fat, ill, malnourished, and hungry, and go against every Clean & Lean rule there is. I don't know about you, but I don't want to eat anything that's been made in a factory, stripped of its natural goodness, and pumped full of manmade preservatives.

Put simply, the less a food has been tampered with, the better it is for your health, looks, and waistline. Unfortunately, however, just about every-thing from pasta, bread, and yogurt to processed meats (like ham) and cans of ravioli has been processed. Having said that, though, not all processed foods are as bad as each other. White bread, for example, has been stripped of all its goodness and pumped full of salt, whereas a pot of organic natural yogurt with just a few ingredients is—while still processed—much better for you because it has retained a lot of its natural goodness. Equally, an organic pasta sauce made mostly of tomatoes is better than a sweet-and-sour flavored sauce containing about ten ingredients, all with scary-sounding names. So when it comes to processed food, just remember: the less that's been done to it the better, and the fewer ingredients it has the better.

The following are the worst processed foods:

- Canned foods
- White bread, pasta, and rice
- Processed meats
- Breakfast cereals
- Frozen meals
- Frozen french fries
- Packages of dried pasta
- Packaged cakes, cookies, muffins
- Chocolate, candy, and potato chips

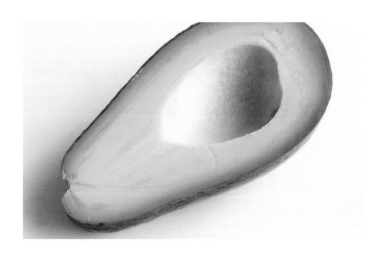

Always check food labels, as although trans fats are now less widely used, they can still be found in the following:

▶ Anything that includes the words "hydrogenated" or "partially hydrogenated" in the ingredients list
▶ Low-fat dairy products
▶ Margarines
▶ Doughnuts, cookies, muffins
▶ Processed meats
▶ Ice cream
▶ Salad dressings
▶ Prepared meals

Processed foods first became really big in the 1970s, when food manufacturers (yes, them again) realized that if they mass produced food that could last a long time it would lead to increased profits. It's much cheaper for them to take poor-quality food, process it, add tons of sugar or sweeteners to flavor and color it, and use a preserving method to lengthen its natural life, than it is for them to use fresh, good-quality ingredients that will spoil after a few days.

One of the most common methods of preserving processed food is to heat it to extreme temperatures, meaning that valuable vitamins, fiber and minerals are lost. That's why fresh fruit is much healthier for you than canned. Remember what I said in Chapter 1—the more vitamins and minerals a food contains, the more it nourishes your body and the less your body will crave sugar and feel hungry. If you never eat anything but processed food, your body is likely to become toxic, you'll never feel satisfied with what you eat, and you'll get cravings. In other words, a toxic body will feel hungry and cling to fat. Studies also suggest that preservatives—found in nearly all processed foods—are likely to slow down metabolism and interfere with fat-burning hormones.

As well as reducing the nutritional value of food, processing has other health implications. Flavorings, colorings, and texture-enhancing agents are added to foods to make them prettier and more appealing. But in some cases these additives can be harmful. Trans fats (see pp. 62–3)—added into things like store-bought muffins and cookies, to extend their shelf life— are one of the worst offenders. Their attraction to manufacturers are obvious, yet trans fats have been linked to infertility, certain cancers, and heart disease and should, as such, be avoided at all costs. Following pressure from health campaigners, food manufacturers are starting to sit up and listen, and trans fats are now being removed from many processed foods. They're still out there though—in a frightening number of foods— so look out for them and give them a very wide berth.

To help you negotiate the minefield, overleaf is my "Bad, Better and Best" guide to processed foods.

Bad	Better	Best
Prepackaged cakes—these sit on the shelves for months with as much nutritional value as the box they come in; stay away from them	A freshly made cake from a baker—a step in the right direction, but still loaded with wheat, sugar, and yeast	Wheat-free, sugar-free, dairy-free muffin from a health-food shop—you'll get fiber and a natural sweetener in the form of fruit
Prepackaged crêpes—white flour and white sugar packed with preservatives; a fat bomb, waiting to explode	Homemade pancakes—better than store-bought, but try to replace white flour with either rice or buckwheat flour	Bodyism pancakes (see p. 77 for recipe) with berries and banana—more easily digested and taste great
Regular chewing gum—too sugary, plus it tells your stomach to "prepare for food," thus giving you a false appetite. Want fresh breath? Why not just brush your teeth!	Sugar- and aspartame-free gum—a little better, but still sending false signals to your brain and stomach	Chew on fresh mint or parsley; herbs are nature's medicine and these will leave your mouth fresh and your body healthy
Packaged meal with no protein (e.g. an all-pasta dish); this will be packed with bad carbs, sugar, salt, and bad fats, as well as leaving you hungry soon after because of the lack of protein	Packaged meal with protein (e.g. chicken or fish)—a step in the right direction, but remember, most meats in these meals are heavily processed and packed with preservatives	A fresh (not frozen or canned) packaged meal with meat, vegetables, and nuts or seeds that can be steamed—not easy to find, but when you absolutely have no time or energy to make food, this is by far the best choice
Salami—the leftover parts of the animal, this is heavily processed and packed with salt, delivering very few nutrients	Slice of ham—at least you know what animal it is!	Ham with hummus and avocado—a complete snack of protein, carbs, and fats
Packaged salad—often dipped in chlorine to retain the color and sprayed with preservatives to give it a long shelf life; don't be fooled by its appearance—this food is nutritionally dead!	Plastic wrapped vegetable, e.g. cucumber; but avoid it where you can and grab the unwrapped stuff	Raw, unpackaged vegetable; this has not gone through a factory and no plastic toxins have leached into it
Salad dressing—packed with sugar, salt, and bad fats	Balsamic vinegar and olive oil—provides a great clean and lean flavor and good fats that help fill you up, making it a more complete dish	Cold-pressed extra virgin olive oil—the least processed of all oils with the most nutrients and the most flavor; or use Udo's essential oil
Water crackers—thin, dead, baked pieces of white flour	Spelt crackers—wheat-free and usually topped with seeds, making a much better dipping cracker	Oatcakes with avocado and smoked salmon—a complete meal with quality protein and good fat

Bad	Better	Best
All sweet crackers (most crackers on the shelf)—loaded with sugar, wheat, bad fats, yeast, with a pinch of salt; need I say more?	Rye crispbread with cheese—wheat-free alternative with a little protein	Oatcakes with avocado and ham—a complete meal with quality protein and good fats
Pretzels—salted wheat; will leave you hungry and thirsty	Organic oven-baked potato chips (the plain ones)—less salt and usually less-bad fats; still not great though	Organic corn chips with guacamole—a wheat-free snack served with good fats, making a much better option
Canned soup	Cardboard or plastic carton of soup	Organic soup with some protein in it, e.g. chicken soup
White pepper	Cracked black pepper	Organic ocean sea salt—contains 82 health-boosting mineral elements
Ketchup	Pesto	Fresh mashed avocado
English mustard	Sweet chili sauce	Garlic paste

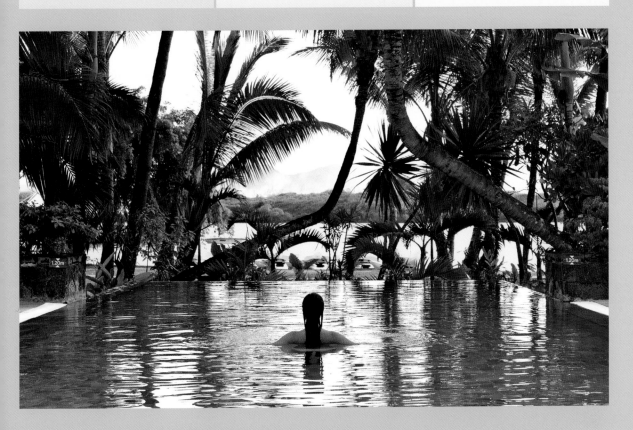

Don't be fooled by food labels

Processed foods sell well because of the clever marketing campaigns behind them. Phrases like "farm fresh," alongside pictures of lush green scenery, kid us into believing that a mass-produced food product made in a factory, using additives and preservatives, has come to us straight from the farm. We need to wise up, and not be fooled by the following:

Ethnic references

Tortilla wraps with Mexican flags on the package, for example, aren't necessarily made in Mexico. They are just there to make you think the food is exotic. It's more likely that they were made in a factory thousands of miles away from Mexico, using cheap white flour and other additives. And the same goes for curry sauces that make references to India.

Healthy claims

Be wary of products that claim to be low-fat, high-fiber or reduced-sugar because there are no legal specifications for these claims. So if a product is labeled low-fat, it just means it has less fat than the standard version of the same product—it doesn't mean it's actually low in fat. The other problem is that if something is marketed as low-fat, it's often high in sugar, which is even worse. Processed cereals are a good example—yes, they're marketed as "low-fat" or "high-fiber," but food manufacturers add extra sugar to make them more palatable.

"Fruit flavor" drinks

There is probably no fruit in these. A drink or yogurt may be labeled as "strawberry flavor" without having to contain any strawberries. However—and this is where it gets confusing—if it's described as "strawberry flavored" (i.e. with an "ed" on the end), then most of the flavor has to come from real strawberries. It will still be heavily processed though, so stick to drinks described as "pure fruit juice" or just squeeze your own juices at home with a juicer.

Emotive descriptions

What do words like "ocean fresh," "country style" and "farm style" really mean? Absolutely nothing, so ignore them.

Healthy ingredients

A product says it contains goji berries or pomegranate, does it? Well, check the ingredients list—you may find it only contains a tiny amount of these ingredients, with a lot of processed sugar coming higher up the ingredients list.

What about processed carbs?

I'm not a fan of low-carb or no-carb diets. However, I do ask my clients to avoid processed carbs, which means most breads, pasta, and rice. Carbs are fine—I eat them all the time—but only in their most natural state, which means vegetables and fruit. There are some processed carbs that are OK—oatcakes, for example, or certain clean, lean breads, like rye. There are so many healthier alternatives to regular bread out there. So instead of white, brown, or multigrain bread (all of which contain lots of wheat; see below for why this is bad), try rice cakes, rye bread, sourdough bread, corn bread, or rice bread instead. Look for them in the health-food section at the supermarket or, better still, at your local health-food shop. And remember always to have protein with your carbs—even good carbs are still fairly high in sugar, so it's important to have some protein with them to slow the rate at which the sugar hits your bloodstream.

And can I eat pasta?

Pasta is incredibly high in wheat (see below), so it can make you fat, sluggish, and bloated. Don't be fooled by wholewheat pastas either—they contain just as much wheat.

If you really love your pasta, look for the following alternatives: vegetable pasta, rice pasta, corn pasta, millet pasta, spelt pasta, buckwheat noodles, or quinoa.

Avoid Wheat—Especially Breakfast Cereals

Throughout this chapter I've mentioned "wheat-free" this and "wheat-free" that. But what's so bad about wheat?

Well, wheat and wheat products (found in so many processed foods) convert to sugar faster than any other grain. And don't forget, sugar converts to fat, so the wheat you eat will very quickly end up as fat all over your hips, thighs, bottom, and stomach. Most breads, pasta, and breakfast cereal consist mainly of wheat, which is why you need to limit them if you want to get a lean and lovely looking body.

Wheat also contains phytates. Phytates bind with health-boosting calcium, iron, magnesium, phosphorus, and zinc in the intestinal tract, preventing these minerals from being properly absorbed. If you eat wheat excessively, you could end up with mineral deficiencies (which make you hungry all the time), allergies (hay fever, skin rashes, and so on), and intestinal problems (such as IBS and bloating).

Nearly all products that contain wheat also contain gluten. Gluten is used mainly as a binder in the processing of food. Without added gluten, ketchup, for example, would be a runny tomato juice. Gluten can be very hard to digest though, and can in susceptible people cause indigestion, yeast overgrowth (candida), allergies, and celiac disease (a digestive disorder that affects the small intestine, causing bloating, diarrhea, constipation, and fatigue).

Do wheat and gluten agree with you?

If your stomach bloats out just below your belly button, especially after

Where's the wheat?

By cutting out wheat and gluten and all foods containing them, you'll lose weight and your stomach will become beautifully flat. However, it's hard to avoid them completely, so just do your best by buying whole, fresh, clean foods and avoiding the following:

All commercial breads	preservatives	Couscous	Puddings containing grain
All commercial breakfast cereals	Canned vegetables (unless canned in water)	Curry powder and seasoning mixes	(stabilizers made from gluten)
Pasta	Cookies	Horseradish creams/sauces	Salad dressings
Muffins	Croissants	Ketchup	Sausages
Pastries	Bagels	Processed meats	Semolina
Baked goods	Alcohol made from grains—	Margarine	Commercially prepared soups
Pizza bases	i.e. beer, whiskey, bourbon	Monosodium glutamate	Soy sauce and most Chinese
Pie crusts	and liqueurs	(MSG—found in many	sauces
Cakes	Cheese spreads	fast foods)	White pepper in restaurants
Canned meat containing	Chewing gum	Mustards	

eating—what I call a "pooch tummy"—this is a classic sign of a wheat or gluten intolerance. Even very slim people get a little pooch tummy that sticks out if they're intolerant to wheat and gluten.

Why you need a wheat-free breakfast (most days)

For many of us, having wheat for breakfast is just a habit. There's no real reason to have toast or cereal first thing, yet so many of us do it out of sheer habit. I tell my clients to have something different—like half an avocado sliced on a few oatcakes. And more often than not, they'll look at me quizzically and say something along the lines of "Are you crazy?" Yet it's so much better for you to have a beautiful, creamy, clean avocado on a crunchy oatcake than a bowl of sugary, salty, processed cereal.

And another great reason to ditch your regular toast or cereal: if you start having wheat-free breakfasts, you could be well on your way to having a lovely, flat stomach.

What's so wrong with breakfast cereals?

The majority of breakfast cereals (with a few exceptions) are far too high in sugar and salt, and are so heavily processed they could even be the C in CRAP. Check out the ingredients label of any breakfast cereal—sugar is often high up in the ingredients list, and this is the last thing you want at breakfast time. Why? Because it will cause a sharp increase in your blood-sugar levels. This, in turn, will increase the production of insulin, which will prevent you from burning fat and encourage your body to store it instead.

Something else worth noting is that cattle are fed on cereal because it's cheap and increases their body weight. Think about it: do you want to start your day with cattle feed?

Even cereals marketed as healthy options aren't what they seem. So ignore the ad of the girl in the swimsuit, or the sports star who tells you he never starts the day without them (I don't believe for a moment an athlete would eat cereal—for one thing, their trainers wouldn't let them, if they're anything like me!) and just check out the ingredients. If wheat, salt, or sugar are on the list, put the box back on the shelf. Stick to lean breakfast foods like eggs, salmon, or avocado instead.

My "Bad, Better and Best" guide to carbs follows on the next page:

Bad	Better	Best
White flour—stripped of all nutrients, white flour also depletes the body of vitamin B	Whole wheat flour—slightly less processed and more fiber, however still contains gluten	Any gluten-free flour—corn flour, rice flour, buckwheat, or millet
White bread	Whole wheat bread	Rye bread
Wheat-based cereal	Oat-based muesli mix with nuts	Half an avocado on a couple of wheat-free oatcakes
Wheat-based white pasta (most pastas)	Whole wheat pasta	Rice and millet, corn, vegetable, or spelt pasta (gluten-free)
Cheese and ham croissant	Bagel with meat and salad	Wheat-free wrap with meat and salad
Store-bought low-fat (and therefore high-sugar) muffin	Oat-based muffin	Sugar-free muffin from a health-food shop
Premade sandwich from shop made with white bread	Rye bread sandwich	One slice of rye bread with extra sandwich filling (tuna, chicken, or meat)
Tortilla—e.g. a burrito	Hard-shell taco	Extra meat filling and salad—no taco
English muffin	Wholegrain/multigrain bread	Rye bread
Doughnuts	Fruit and nut butter	Fruit and nuts
Pasta dish	Bolognese sauce with rice	Super Ground Beef (see p. 98) with brown rice
Couscous—too processed	White rice	Brown rice
Jasmine/white rice	Basmati rice	Brown/wild rice
Packaged waffles (full of sugar, salt, and all kinds of other junk)	Freshly made waffles	Bodyism pancakes (see p. 77 for the recipe)
Scones, jam, and cream	Scones and organic cream (no jam)	Bran muffin with organic butter
Cookies	Rice cakes with nut butter	Rice cakes with avocado and shrimp

Bad	Better	Best
Potato chips	Kettle chips	Salted celery with hummus
Pizza bases	Whole wheat pizza base	Wheat-free pizza base, e.g. spelt
Jam or cranberry condiment	Honey	Organic nut butter, e.g. hazel, cashew, almond, peanut
Peanut butter (commercial), made with roasted, salted peanuts	Unsalted peanut butter	Organic nut butter, e.g. almond, cashew, and macadamia
Fries	Thick-sliced potato wedges	Baked potato with some protein (shrimp, hummus)
An apple Danish	A handful of dried apple	A handful of sliced fresh apple with almonds
Crackers	Rice cakes	Rice or oatcakes with protein, e.g. hummus
Store-bought cake	Fresh cake from a good-quality baker	Homemade cake, made with fruit as the sweetener and no white sugar
Canned fruit	Peeled fruit	Whole fruit (the skin contains most of the fiber)
Cereal breakfast bars	Banana	Banana and a handful of nuts
Canned vegetables	Frozen vegetables	Fresh organic vegetables
Stewed fruit	Peeled fruit	Whole organic fruit

Remember! Food manufacturers will try to trick you by using less obvious names for wheat, such as corn starch, edible starch, food starch, modified starch, rusk, thickener, or vegetable protein.

Chapter 4
Why Stress Makes You Fat

This chapter will reveal…

▶ How destressing can make you slim

▶ Why too much exercise can make you fat

▶ Why how you eat is as important as what you eat

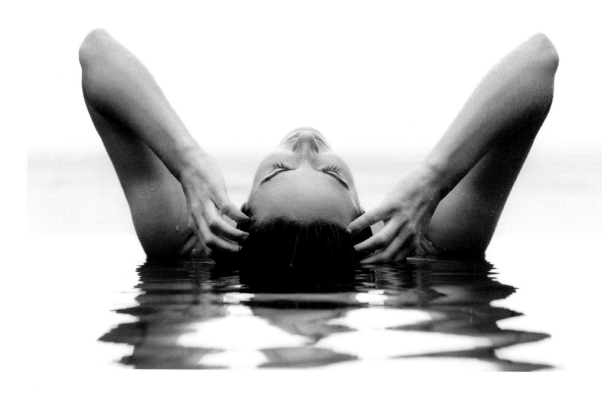

How Destressing Can Make You Slim

Aside from alcohol, too much coffee, and bad food, stress is one of the biggest causes of excess fat. If you're doing everything else correctly (avoiding sugar, eating good fat, etc.), but you're stressed, you will still have a fat little tummy and a thick waist.

When we're frightened, angry, tense, or worried, our bodies become flooded with adrenaline and a stress hormone called cortisol (released from our adrenal glands—a tiny gland that sit just above our kidneys.) The adrenaline keeps us alert and focused, while the cortisol prepares our muscles for a "fight-or-flight" response. It's actually known as the "fight-or-flight" hormone because it gives us an immediate burst of energy that we can use either to "fight," i.e. confront a potentially harmful situation, or for "flight," i.e. to run away from it. It also helps the body to release sugar into the bloodstream for instant energy.

That sickly, jittery, panicky feeling you get in the pit of your stomach when you are stressed comes from the adrenaline and cortisol. It's all part of a defence mechanism that allows the body to respond appropriately when faced with danger and that was designed to keep us out of harm's way (especially in cavemen times when we had to run away from all kinds of dangerous animals).

Why modern stress is bad for you

While the stress mechanism worked well for us when we were cavemen, modern-day stress is not so good.

In fact, modern stress, caused by a relentlessly busy lifestyle, is really, really bad for you—even toxic. It causes you to get fat (I'll explain why below), it wears out your immune system, and it increases your risk of serious illness. This is because many of the situations that cause you to become stressed nowadays aren't the sort of danger that you need to run away from—although your body still wants you to. While an important job interview, a looming deadline, or being told off by a scary boss may feel frightening, they won't cause you any physical harm, so there is no need for you to run away from them—which brings me to why stress makes you fat.

Why stress makes you fat

We've established that when you get stressed your body releases adrenaline and cortisol, and that when you're in real (i.e. physical) danger, these hormones prompt you either to run away or fight, in which case they don't make you fat. But when you're not in real danger, you don't use these fat-storing hormones, so they—and all that sugar that is released into the bloodstream—just float around, eventually ending up as fat on your tummy and around your waist. They also make you crave more sugar (in the form of chocolate and cookies) because your body thinks it needs more to keep it going. This is why stressed people often lose a couple of pounds on vacation—even though they may be eating the same amount as usual or sometimes even more, they don't have fat-storing hormones floating around their system every day, high blood-sugar levels, or constant cravings.

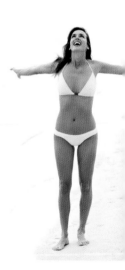

The stress hormone cortisol is particularly bad for you because studies show it's directly related to abdominal fat. As stress levels subside, your adrenaline levels fall, but cortisol (and the resulting blood sugar) stays in the system much longer. Research shows that fat cells around the stomach area attract cortisol, giving you a layer of toxic fat just below your abdominal muscles that's really hard to shift. So doing regular sit-ups is going to be pointless if you always feel stressed—the only way to ditch this fat is to ditch the stress in your life. And remember—stomach fat is the most dangerous type of fat there is because it raises your risk of heart disease, high blood pressure, diabetes, and certain cancers.

Why stress makes you ill

As we've seen, the adrenal glands are the ones that release cortisol into the system. In many of my clients, these glands are overworked, making them unwell and overweight. Remember, they are meant for emergencies—like encounters with crazy animals or strangers in alleys; they're not meant to be worked every single day. Yet many of my clients—probably like many of you—live in a world of constant, low-level, unrelenting stress: they oversleep; they rush around getting their kids (or themselves) ready for the day; they run out of the house with only coffee to keep them going (remember—coffee also causes your system to become stressed); then they face a day of late buses, traffic jams, deadlines, long lines, annoying colleagues, and so on. All day long, their bodies are being flooded with adrenaline, and their poor, overworked adrenals are secreting cortisol to help them deal with all the stressful situations they find themselves in. They're literally running on empty, and their systems begin to break down. Overworked adrenal glands can cause lowered immunity (resulting in constant colds and illnesses), tiredness, and fatigue. Sleep is affected, too (if you've ever tried to fall asleep while the next day's to-do list is racing around in your mind, you'll know how true this is). Constant stress also shuts down the digestive system because your body redirects blood from there (namely to your muscles). So stress can leave you constipated, bloated, and toxic. Beating this stress is the only way to better health and a better body.

Why some foods make you more stressed

It's not just stress that makes you stressed—the wrong type of food does too. Potentially toxic foods—like refined sugar and processed foods (see Chapters 2 and 3)—will make you feel more stressed because they release sugar into the bloodstream too quickly. This increases the amount of stress in your body and also allows too much insulin into your system, which, in turn, plays a huge role in fat storage by making it harder for your body to burn off fat. Together, too much insulin and cortisol combine to give you a double whammy of fat storage plus increased appetite. It's a vicious cycle—the more stressed you get, the more you crave toxic food, which makes you more stressed, and so the cycle continues.

Clean, lean foods, on the other hand, give you long-lasting energy, thus reducing stress levels. So break the cycle. Just chill out, don't exercise too much (see p. 52), avoid stress-inducing foods, and eat more stress-reducing ones (see p.50).

Remember! When under attack from stress, your adrenal glands also produce DHEA (dehydroepiandrosterone), which converts into estrogen, progesterone, and testosterone. That's why too much stress has a major effect on your sex hormones and can lead to a lower sex drive and fertility problems.

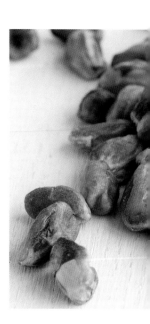

Stress-inducing foods

Candy—sugary snacks give you a quick burst of energy, but then cause your blood-sugar levels to crash, leaving you feeling sluggish, stressed, and with poor concentration. Avoid them like the plague.

Processed foods—these are full of junk and deplete the levels of vitamins and minerals in your body, leaving you more prone to stress. Stick to clean, lean, natural foods.

Junk food—studies show that foods high in bad fats (burgers, fries, chicken nuggets, etc.) lower your concentration levels and increase your stress levels. Hence that tired, jittery, weird feeling you get after a bag of greasy junk food.

Salty foods—these increase your blood pressure, making you more prone to stress. The worst offenders are processed meats like ham and bacon, and processed foods that are stuffed with salt.

Coffee—as I explained in Chapter 3, too much caffeine stresses out your system by constantly flooding your body with the fat-storing hormone cortisol. Stick to one or two cups of organic coffee a day.

Alcohol—this stimulates your poor, overworked adrenal glands. If you have a stressful life and you drink a lot, your adrenal glands will be exhausted. Go easy on alcohol to give them a chance to recover. Alcohol is also full of sugar, which makes you toxic and fat. People mistakenly think it will help them to unwind after a hard day, but it has the opposite effect—it just stresses your whole system further. If you really can't do without, see p. 35 for advice.

Stress-reducing foods

Berries—these are packed with vitamin C, which helps the body to deal with stress. Plus, they're full of fiber which helps to regulate blood-sugar levels. (Remember—blood-sugar levels fluctuate when you're stressed.) Have a handful of berries with your breakfast.

Green vegetables—dark green vegetables help to replenish the body with vitamins in times of stress. Have these with every meal if you can (even breakfast!), but make sure they're organic.

Turkey—this contains an amino acid called L-tryptophan, which releases serotonin (a calming, feel-good hormone) into the body. Eating turkey has a soothing effect on the body and can even help you sleep better. Keep it clean and lean by choosing skinless and organic turkey.

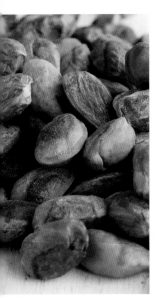

Sweet potatoes—they'll satisfy a carb craving, but contain more fiber and vitamins than white potatoes.

Avocados—they're creamy, so they satisfy cravings. Plus, all the good fat and potassium they contain can lower your blood pressure (and therefore stress levels). Have half an avocado on its own as a snack or with oatcakes for a delicious stress-busting breakfast.

Nuts—they help boost a battered immune system, plus they're full of B vitamins, which help to lower stress levels. Snack on a small handful, but don't go overboard with your portion sizes. Stick to a handful a day.

Bodyism bodySerenity—this formula, sold at my gym and online, has essential minerals and vitamins, such as magnesium, to aid restful sleep, and it can reduce cortisol levels before sleep.

Bodyism bodyBrilliance—a stress-busting blend of vitamins, minerals, fiber, and protein, this is one of the best ways to kickstart your day.

TOM AND GRACE'S STORY

When Tom and his wife Grace came to see me, Tom was overworked and unwell. He was also fat, fragile, and defeated. He had worked himself into the ground at the office and was overweight, yet undernourished, with a big stomach and sky-high stress levels. Grace was also stressed, but not as much as her husband. As is the case with a lot of new clients, they were deeply cynical and thought they knew best. When I explained my Clean & Lean approach, they said they'd try it for a week and "see how things go." I told them that "seeing how things go" never got anybody anywhere and that they needed to commit fully if they wanted to see change. I told them to trust me and follow a few easy steps.

Over the next couple of months, the fat fell off their stomachs and the color came back into their cheeks. Grace had a huge addiction to sugar, which we kicked; she was grumpy at first, but she stuck with it, her skin glowed and she got clean and lean. After two months, Tom had lost 26 pounds and Grace lost 15 pounds. But the best part? After years of trying, Grace became pregnant. Just like that. It's times like those that make me really love my job!

BEN'S STORY

Ben was the most highly strung person I'd ever met. Aged 32, he was a high-flying, high-earning banker who was constantly pushing himself to be better at everything. When he turned up for his first session with me he said, "My assistant told me you're the best. You have six weeks to get this disgusting fat off my stomach." He also told me he'd been to every top gym, trainer, and nutritionist in London, but nothing had worked. He was already running for ten hours a week on a treadmill, but said he'd double that if he had to.

I told Ben that he'd never get the washboard stomach he so badly wanted if he kept stressing out his system. I also told him he needed to stop all that running as he only needed one yoga class a week, plus another two or three sessions with me. Then I looked at his diet, which was full of low-fat rubbish, including "diet" cereals and "diet" cereal bars. I asked him to replace these fat bombs with lots of clean protein (such as organic chicken) and green vegetables. But most importantly, I told him to just chill out.

To his credit, Ben did everything I told him, and four weeks after first walking through my door, he had a six pack. All his happy eating and chilling meant his body wasn't storing fat—it was shedding it. His only complaint was that he'd become less scary at work, which wasn't good for his reputation as a man to be feared!

Why Too Much Exercise Can Make You Fat

I see lots of high-flying business people who are literally running themselves fat on the treadmill. Why? Because if exercising makes you stressed—either because you're doing too much of it or because you're running around to squeeze your gym classes in after work—then it might also be making you fat because of all the extra cortisol you're producing.

People who go to the gym too often can still have slightly pudgy stomachs, even when the rest of their body is well sculpted. If new clients tells me (proudly) that they go to the gym five or six times a week, I tell them to cut it down to twice or three times and to replace a cardio session (e.g. a run on the treadmill) with a yoga or Pilates session to calm them down and relax their system (see Chapter 9 for more on Clean & Lean exercise).

Why *How* You Eat Is As Important As *What* You Eat

You can follow all the diet and exercise rules in this book to the letter, but if you're skipping meals, eating too quickly, or eating while stressed, you'll never be clean and lean.

One of the best things you can do for your body is to learn how to chew properly. Chewing is the cornerstone of healthy eating. A salad, for example, is not really that healthy unless you chew it properly. This is because chewing food releases all the vitamins and minerals contained in the food. Chewing also produces saliva and breaks down food, so it can be more easily digested after you've swallowed it. And well-digested food can help give you a flat stomach and a healthy body. If you eat too fast and swallow half-chewed lumps of food, they'll fester in your stomach and take longer to digest, resulting in bloating and gas.

What I want you to do is to take your time over every single meal. It should take you at least—at least—twenty minutes to finish a meal. More if it's a big meal. I want you to chew every single mouthful at least—at least—twenty times. More if you can manage it. I want you to chew each mouthful of food until it's a watery, mushy paste. And I promise this will have an amazing effect on your body.

ZOE'S STORY

"I used to be the queen of quick eating, but learning to chew has given me a flat stomach. I used to eat breakfast at my desk, which would usually be muesli that I would swallow half chewed. I'd often be so busy I'd eat lunch at 3 p.m., by which point I'd be ravenous. I'd grab a sandwich and eat it in less than 10 minutes before racing off to a meeting. I'd grab snacks all afternoon and eat them quickly, too. Then, when I got home, I'd be in such a rush for food that I'd swallow down mouthfuls of pasta that I hadn't even chewed properly. I always felt bloated, and my stomach stuck out like I was in the early stages of pregnancy.

James has taught that no matter how busy you are, you can always put aside 20 minutes to eat something properly. I started chewing every mouthful thoroughly, which meant I could really taste my food. Within about two weeks, my stomach was completely flat."

How not to stress-eat

- Chew each mouthful at least twenty times—thirty if you can manage it.
- Put your cutlery down and take a few breaths between each mouthful.
- Don't swallow until your food is a watery paste.
- Only ever eat when you're relaxed. If you're stressed, wait until you feel better before eating.
- Stop when you're full, and don't be afraid to leave food on your plate. You can always have more food later on, if you become hungry again.
- Don't mistake stress for hunger—if you're stressed, you need to calm down, not eat.
- Make sure you're drinking plenty of water—when you're stressed it's easy to forget to stay hydrated.
- Don't watch TV or do any type of work while you're eating. Focusing on something other than your food can lead to overeating.

The benefits of eating properly

- Your stress levels will reduce.
- You'll look and feel less bloated.
- You'll feel fuller quicker, so you'll eat less at mealtimes and look leaner.
- You won't feel uncomfortably full or bloated.
- You won't mindlessly munch—when you stress-eat, you don't take time to listen to your body properly, so you often end up eating when you're not even hungry.

What Are You Actually Hungry For?

This is a question I tell clients to ask themselves when they're rooting through the cupboards for something to snack on. And, more often than not, they're not hungry for food; they're looking for a distraction because they're stressed, lonely, bored, or tired. All these emotions make you hungry for something—but food is not the answer.

If you're stressed, you're hungry because your body is flooded with adrenaline and cortisol, which play havoc with your sugar levels, causing you to crave something sweet. But instead of reaching for the cookies, you need to take time out, breathe deeply, and work through your stress before you eat anything. The same goes if you're lonely or bored: find some-thing else to distract yourself with—either a TV show, a movie, or a hot bath. Or you could be proactive with your body and do your 8-minute workout if you get hungry (see p. 120)! Eating won't cheer you up; it'll just provide a short distraction.

If you're tired, allow yourself to be tired. I'm constantly amazed at how many people don't let themselves wind down in the evening—they're always looking for a quick fix to prop up their flagging energy levels after work, whether it's a glass of wine, some chocolate, or a cup of coffee. Allow your body to fall into tiredness and get an early night. Don't prop yourself up with a constant stream of stimulants.

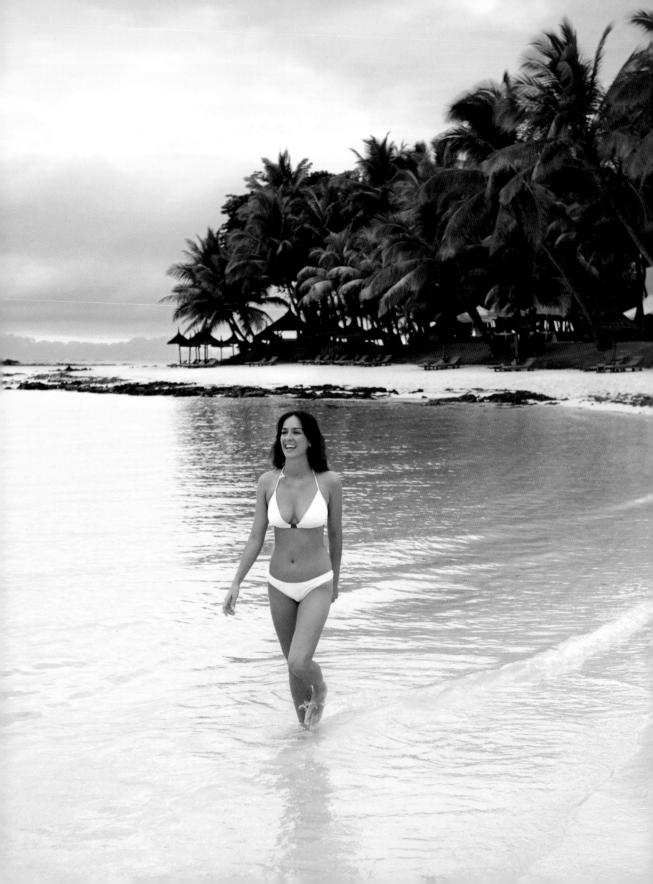

Chapter 5
Why (Good) Fat Makes You Slim

This chapter will reveal...

▸ How fat phobia is ruining your diet

▸ Why (good) fat is so slimming

▸ How to cook fat the Clean & Lean way

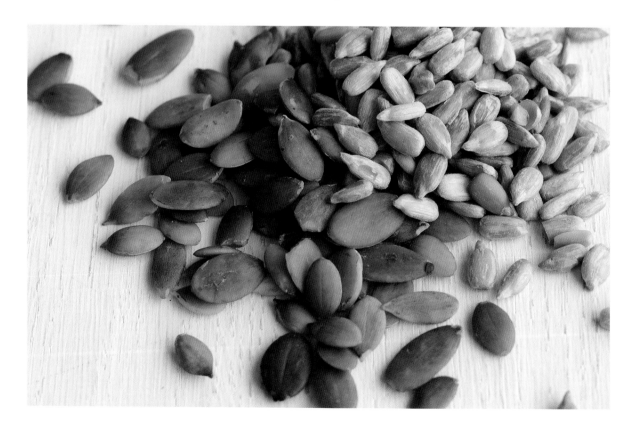

How Fat Phobia is Ruining Your Diet

Growing up, it's drummed into all of us that fat makes us, well, fat, of course. Our moms went on fat-free or low-fat diets when they wanted to lose weight, and we took note. Fat was—and still is—seen as the big bad baddie of food, standing between us and our dream body. Its name alone gives it a bad reputation because it's associated with the fat sitting around our waist (and clinging to our thighs) that we're desperately trying to shift.

But guess what? Fat doesn't make you fat. Sugar does, and so do bad carbs (both of which, ironically, are almost entirely fat-free). But fat? Absolutely not. In fact, eating good fat—as you'll learn in this chapter—will make you very slim indeed. It's like the anti-sugar. In the same way that sugar gives you premature wrinkles, makes you hungry, and causes you to gain weight, good fat will take years off your face, banish your hunger and cravings, and help you whittle down your waist. So don't be afraid of fat. But just to reiterate—I am talking about "good fat" here, not "bad fat." And I'll explain the difference later on in this chapter.

When they first come to see me, nearly all my clients tell me proudly that they have very little fat in their diets. In fact, one of the biggest complaints I hear is: "I just don't get it, James. I have hardly any fat in my diet and buy low-fat or fat-free versions of everything, but I just can't lose weight." And I tell them it's because they don't eat any fat that they are fat. If they'd get over their fat phobia, they'd lose weight.

Why (Good) Fat is So Good

First things first: not all fats are created equal. When I refer to fat, I'm talking about the good type—the type that makes you slim, young-looking and energized. This type of fat is found in foods like nuts, seeds, oils, meat, fish, seafood, and avocados.

Good fat prevents you from overeating by telling your brain when to stop. You literally cannot binge on good fat because it fills you up so much. Don't believe me? Then try having half an avocado on some oatcakes for

HANNAH'S STORY

When twenty-three-year-old Hannah came to see me she couldn't understand why she was a size 12 and tired all the time. She said she went to the gym three times a week, yet couldn't lose weight and was actually slowly putting it on.

When she told me what she ate, it was no surprise to me that she couldn't shift the pounds—she was eating hardly any good fat and surviving on what I call "low-fat fat bombs." I cleaned up her diet immediately and got rid of all the sugar she was eating. And I added some much needed good fat. Within a week, her face was slimmer and her eyes shone. (Your body responds quickly to being cleaned up.) We also cut her gym time in half and created some long, lean muscles with light weights, which fired up her metabolism even further. Within three months, Hannah had dropped from a size 12 to a size 6, and from 150 to 125 pounds. She now eats fat all the time, and looks clean, lean, and lovely.

breakfast—you won't be hungry until lunchtime. Then, the next day, try having some low-fat cereal with skimmed milk and fruit, or some toast and low-fat spread. Chances are you'll be hungry less than two hours later. This is why fat-phobic dieters are hungry all the time (and tired and miserable). There's something in good fat that switches on your brain's "stomach full" signals, and countless studies show that people who eat good fat every day are slimmer than those who don't.

For this reason, I tell all my clients that they must have some fat with every single meal and snack. It goes against a lot of what they thought before, but it works. So never eat anything without having a bit of fat with it: if you have some grapes, eat a few almonds at the same time; if you have a salad, add some avocado or organic goat's cheese, or even just a splash of olive oil. Never have a fat-free salad.

Fat slows the rate at which sugar hits your bloodstream, and this allows your blood-sugar levels to remain steady, keeping hunger and cravings at bay and leaving you slim and energized. So no meal or snack should ever be totally fat-free. I know I'm repeating myself here, but I can't stress enough how great you'll look and feel when you start introducing good fat with everything.

Good fat also burns fat and gives you a flat stomach and a small waist. Essential fatty acids—found in oily fish like salmon—help to shift fat out of the fat cells and into the bloodstream where it can be worked off by the body. Studies also show that these fatty acids help the body burn fat around the midsection—basically, your waist and stomach—which is most people's trouble spot. I've often noticed that people who stick to a very low-fat diet tend to be a bit thicker around the middle, no matter how little they weigh. So always pick the full-fat version when you're choosing what to eat; choose butter over margarine and regular hummus over the so-called "diet" version. Not only will the full-fat products make you cleaner and keep you fuller for longer, but the "low-fat" options are usually pumped full of toxic, processed, low-calorie sugar, salt, and sweeteners.

Most people overeat "low-fat" diet products, too, because they are lulled by them into a false sense of security. When you're eating low-fat hummus, for example, it's tempting to polish off half a container because there's a great big sticker on the package reminding you that it's "reduced fat" or "lite." Equally, when you're adding margarine to your baked potato, it's easy to slather on a ton of it because it's "low-fat." Also, low-fat products often don't contain as much flavor. For example, butter contains something called CLA, which is great for fat burning, plus it enhances the

MANDY'S STORY

Mandy, a thirty-four-year-old mother of two, was a financial executive and super-stressed. She told me she had tried literally everything to lose weight; she was living on "diet" and low-fat foods but was only getting fatter.

Mandy thought she knew a lot about nutrition and was very strict with herself, but she was getting it hopelessly wrong. For breakfast she'd have a bowl of supposedly healthy breakfast cereal. Then she'd have diet cereal bars, diet cola, and coffee for the rest of the time. Her diet may have been lean, but it certainly wasn't clean.

The first thing I did was to halve her exercise load. She was in the gym all the time, stressing her body out and making it produce extra cortisol, which was depositing fat all over her tummy. The next thing I did was to get her off all the diet junk she was hooked on. Within a week she'd lost 5 pounds, even though she wasn't exercising as much and was eating more fat. It only took six weeks to get Mandy completely clean and lean, from a size 14 to a size 8 and 20 pounds lighter.

flavor of food making it richer, so satisfying your appetite in a way that a low-fat spread never will. I'd much rather my clients put a little bit of organic butter on their food (which is all they need to keep their taste buds happy), rather than smothering it with a toxic, processed, low-fat spread that will never, ever satisfy them.

Good fat also helps your body to absorb vitamins and minerals better. Take a salad, for example—if you eat it on its own, you'll still get all the benefits from all those great vegetables, but it might leave you feeling a bit unsatisfied and hungry an hour or so later. But if you add some fat to it—say, half an avocado or a drizzle of olive oil—your body will be able to absorb the nutrients much better. And remember—as I explained earlier—a body full of nutrients doesn't feel hungry; it burns fat a lot quicker and it doesn't feel tired (so doesn't need to snack on toxic sugar to keep it going). Adding fat to a salad also makes it more satisfying, so you'll feel full hours after eating it and won't need to snack as much.

Another advantage of good fat is that it helps to cushion your joints from wear and tear. If you exercise, you absolutely have to have some fat in your diet to prevent injuries. It also boosts your concentration and energy levels, plus it gives you amazing-looking hair, skin, and nails (see p. 112 to find out why a fat-free diet gives you wrinkles).

In my opinion eating enough good fat also banishes the following (all-too-common) problems:

- Inability to concentrate
- Sluggishness
- Feeling physically full, but still hungry (i.e. that feeling you get when you're hungry shortly after a meal)
- Craving something sweet after food
- A sudden mid-afternoon energy drop
- Difficulty waking up in the morning
- A feeling of lethargy and fatigue

How to eat fat

For a start, you need to know the difference between good (clean) fat and bad (toxic) fat. Good fat is monounsaturated fat (MUFA), and it's found mainly in nuts, avocados, and olive oil. It helps to lower bad cholesterol and reduces

How to choose a supplement
There are so many fish oil supplements on the market—some are high quality, and some aren't. A good way of testing any kind of pill or supplement is to leave it in a glass of water overnight. A good-quality pill will break down and dissolve—a bad one won't, which implies that when you take it, it's going straight through you.

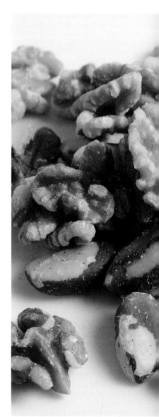

overall body fat by revving up your metabolism. Then there's polyunsaturated fat, which also lowers bad cholesterol levels and is found mainly in fish and seafood. As I've said before, a meal or snack is not complete (or healthy), unless it has a bit of fat with it, so see my Clean & Lean fat lists below.

I tell my clients to take a fish oil (omega 3) supplement, too. Wherever she is in the world, Elle take fish oils every day and I always say, if you don't take any other supplements, then at least take these. They top up levels of essential fatty acids and also encourage your body to burn fat (around your stomach and waist in particular), plus they boost energy levels and improve your skin. Bodyism Fish Oil sold at my gym and online has been certified to contain no toxic chemicals or additives at all.

The following fish aren't oily or as rich in omega 3 fatty acids, but they're still incredibly healthy. Cod is also fantastic for you, but it's massively over-fished at the moment, so avoid it if you can.

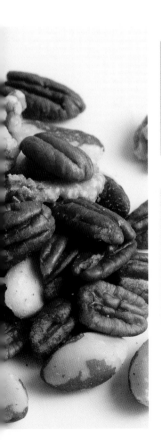

Clean & Lean nuts and seeds

- Almonds
- Pecans
- Walnuts
- Brazil nuts
- Pistachios

- Macadamias
- Cashews
- Chestnuts
- Sesame seeds
- Peanuts

- Sunflower seeds
- Pumpkin seeds
- Flax seed (ground only)

Clean & Lean seafood

The following are all rich in fatty acids:

- Salmon*
- Trout
- Striped bass
- Mackerel*
- Anchovies
- Herring
- Sardines
- Catfish
- Perch

- Tuna* (go for fresh steaks or the kind in glass jars— these are available in health-food shops or delis)
- Swordfish*
- Lemon sole
- Haddock
- Monkfish
- Bluefish

- Red snapper
- Flounder
- Skate
- Halibut
- Dover sole
- Red and gray mullet
- Sea bass
- Sea bream
- Lobster

*These fish contain mercury, so limit yourself to two or three servings a week (or, if you're pregnant, just one or two servings a week). *Note:* see my fish recipes in Chapter 7.

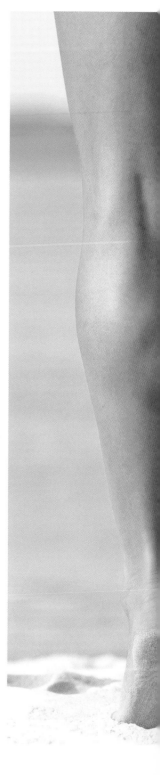

> ## Clean & Lean oils for cooking
>
> **When cooking on a medium heat:**
>
> • Macadamia nut oil   • Avocado oil
>
> **When cooking on a high heat:**
>
> • Ghee (clarified butter)   • Coconut oil
>
> *Note:* Don't cook with olive oil—believe it or not, cold olive oil is a healthy fat full of goodness. But heated up, it becomes a bad fat. Olive oil breaks down at high temperatures and becomes more carcinogenic (i.e. toxic). Only ever use olive oil cold as a salad dressing or heat it up gently for short periods (say, if you're stir-frying shrimp or vegetables for a few minutes).

Bad fats

There are a few bad types of fat that give all the other fats a bad name. Trans fats are the worst (see also p. 37) and are found in nearly all processed foods. Food manufacturers created trans fats (basically, a nasty reheated oil) to prolong their products' shelf life and add flavor. Fresh, clean, organic food spoils very quickly because it contains nothing unnatural or toxic to preserve it, but food that contains trans fats lasts for ages (think of those muffins that survive in sweaty plastic wrappers for months on end—yuck). A good rule of thumb is to eat only foods that go off after a few days.

Trans fats are associated with some of the scariest health risks of all the fats. They've been linked to obesity, some cancers, and even infertility. People who eat trans fats have higher blood levels of interleukin-6, which, research shows, increases your risk of heart disease, and can also reduce muscle tone and metabolism.

Some states and cities have banned trans fats from restaurants. They are seriously bad news—even worse than saturated fat (see opposite page)—and you should avoid them at all costs. The worst offenders are some processed cookies, muffins, margarines, pastries, and potato chips, but they can also be found in diet foods, mousses, protein shakes and bars, and just about anything with a long shelf life. Food manufacturers don't always list trans fats as such on their ingredients lists because they know they've got such a bad reputation; avoid "hydrogenated oil," "hydrogenated vegetable fat," and "partially hydrogenated vegetable oil," which are trans fats hiding under a different name.

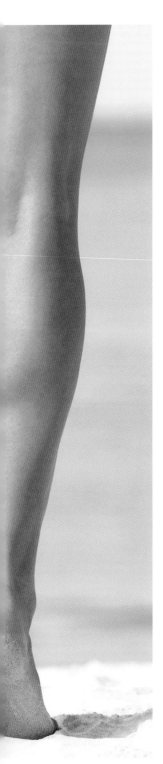

Then there is saturated fat. This isn't as bad as trans fat, because it's natural. But it's still fattening, so it's best to avoid it where possible and only indulge occasionally. Often called "sat fat" on food packages, this raises bad cholesterol levels and is found mainly in animal products like meat and full-fat dairy.

Here's my quick at-a-glance guide to bad fat:

Anything with a crust—next time you order a pie, take off the pastry and enjoy the filling.

Pizza—most packaged pizzas are layer upon layer of wheat (which converts to fat), topped with cheese that's processed and laced with additives. The actual topping—the chicken and mushrooms, for example—make up a tiny percentage of the whole pizza.

Prepared meals—you can find bad fat in practically every single packaged food. Just make your own meal—it takes a little longer, but it'll make you cleaner and leaner.

Olive oil—if heated to high temperatures (see above).

Avoid store-bought cakes—cookies and muffins. Despite what the labels say, they haven't been "home-baked"—they've been processed in a factory and pumped full of junk to keep them "fresh" for as long as possible.

Anything described as deep-fried, sautéed, or breaded.

Any obvious fat on an animal product—for example, the white rind on a slice of bacon. Don't forget, toxins are stored in the fat of animals (as they are in humans), so always cut off the excess fat.

Salad dressings—they're usually high in sugar, salt and trans fats. Add good fat (and clean flavor) to your salad instead by ordering extra avocado or using extra-virgin olive oil. And remember, don't be fooled by a low-fat salad dressing—low fat just means high in sugar, which in turn converts to fat around your waist.

What about dairy?

Almost all my clients ask me about dairy—usually along the lines of, "Will it make me fat?" or, "Will giving it up make me slim?" The answer is that dairy is OK if you're OK with it—if it doesn't make you bloated or uncomfortably full, keep having it. But many people find the lactose in cow's milk hard to digest, so if you're regularly gassy or bloated then you may be intolerant. In which case, reduce the amount you drink or eliminate if from your diet and replace it with more easily digested alternatives like almond, oat, rice, or hazelnut milk.

If you are having milk, use the best you can find. Ideally, this means raw, organic, unpasteurized and unhomogenized milk. Pasteurisation involves heating milk to just below boiling point, a process that kills bacteria but also—crucially for the food manufacturers—extends the shelf life of milk. However, the process also kills off lots of the goodness, and unpasteurised milk has much higher levels of nutrients and omega 3s. As I've been saying all along, the less a food has been tampered with, the better it is. However, unpasteurized milk is fairly controversial—officially it's considered unsafe and in Europe it has to carry a warning to this effect. In fact, it is illegal in Australia and in some parts of the United States. It can therefore be hard to find good-quality, organic unpasteurized milk, but try health-food shops and local organic delis.

Goat's milk is a good alternative to cow's milk. It's actually better for you because it's easier to digest, and it's closer in molecular structure to human breast milk, which your body is designed to handle.

It almost goes without saying that your milk should be organic. If you can't afford much in the way of organic food, just buy organic milk (and meat). Countless studies show that organic milk contains more nutrients than nonorganic, plus it contains omega 3 fatty acids. The same goes for yogurt—forget the low-fat/high-sugar rubbish that's been dyed pink to make you believe it's full of strawberries; just buy organic, full-fat goat's yogurt instead. Low-fat flavored yogurts will make you toxic and fat. Remember: good fat doesn't make you fat—sugar does.

And what about cheese? Well, it's full of saturated fat (see page 63), so it's best eaten in moderation. As a rule, if it's bright yellow and packed in slices, avoid it altogether. (Remember to look beyond the marketing— those "high in calcium" claims on the packet—and a little more carefully at the ingredients. If it contains anything you can't pronounce or understand, ditch it.) A good natural cheese, on the other hand (organic of course), can contain good nutrients and minerals. Try to buy sheep's or goat's cheese as these tend to be a little less processed and better for you. Once you've finished your 14-day Kickstart, you can introduce a little bit of good cheese into your diet.

What's the difference between fat and protein?

Protein is the building block of every hormone and increases your metabolism. Protein is basically anything that used to run, walk, swim, or fly. For example, chicken, eggs (from something that used to walk), fish, shellfish, beef, etc. It's made up of amino acids, which help lay down lean muscle mass, which, as well as giving you the appearance of looking toned, also helps to speed up your metabolism and keep you strong and healthy.

Fat comes in many forms, and there are good and bad fats. The good ones are called essential fatty acids (EFAs)—they're essential because we can't produce them ourselves. Good fats give us a full feeling and are incredibly beneficial for just about every system and process within the body. However, when you eat meat, fat is the white stuff on the edges, and generally the harder the fat, the more full of toxins it is, so trim off the hard fat on the side of meat. Stay away from trans fats—if you see trans fat on the label, put it back on the shelf.

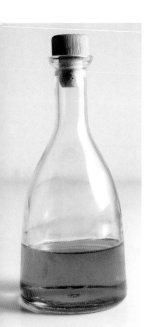

How to Cook Fat the Clean & Lean Way

Here are some tips on keeping your fat as healthy as possible when you're preparing it:

Never, ever microwave your protein. Remember, microwaves kill the goodness in food. With protein, microwaves also alter the molecular structure, leaving it unrecognizable to your gut wall.

Never overcook your meat—the longer it cooks, the more goodness is lost. (Note: always cook chicken thoroughly because it has such a high food-poisoning risk.) Never blacken or char your meat or fish—the black stuff is toxic to your system. Bake or boil (lightly)—you'll retain more of the vitamins.

See my "Bad, Better and Best" guide to fat on the following page. Always try to stay well away from foods in the "Bad" column.

Remember! Try to get all your fat from food or good-quality supplements. Avoid adding it to meals in the form of margarine, mayo, or creamy sauces. If you pick foods that are rich in natural fat (such as eggs, salmon, etc.), you won't need to add more toxic fat. Keep it as clean and as natural as possible.

Bad	Better	Best
Cooking fats: even olive oil, which breaks down easily at high temperatures, making fat rancid	Rapeseed oil	Organic extra-virgin coconut oil—this doesn't break down at high temperatures
Store-bought salad dressing	Extra-virgin olive oil	Organic, cold-pressed extra-virgin olive oil
Margarine	Regular butter	Unsalted raw butter
Hydrogenated/partially hydrogenated oils (trans fats)	Vegetable oil	Fats naturally found in oily fish; salmon, mackerel, albacore tuna, herring, and sardines are the best
Packaged, pre-made guacamole—processed and packed with preservatives and E numbers; usually uses overripe avocados	Homemade guacamole—a better alternative and a really great dip	Bodyism guacamole—packed with good fats, vegetables, antioxidants, and flavor (see p. 94 for the recipe)
Roasted and salted nuts	Raw salted nuts	Raw unsalted nuts
Vegetable-based margarines—soya or sunflower	Organic cow's butter	Organic goat's butter
Doughnuts—the worst of all pastries, packed with additives and sugar that destroy any attempts at fat loss.	Muffin from a health-food shop— it may contain some fiber and fruit (and satisfy your sweet craving), but it's still pumped full of fat and sugar	Fruit and nuts—the perfect mix of fat and good sugar to satisfy your sweet craving and help fill you up; eat the fat (nuts) first.
Croissant—zero-fiber, dead pastry soaked in bad fats	Muffin from health-food shop—see above	Raw vegetables with just a little organic hummus—loads of fiber, vitamins and minerals
Bacon—full of nitrates which drag nutrients from your body, including essential vitamins A, C and E	Ham slices	Organic ham off the bone, in its cleanest, most natural state
Fries/crisps—the thinner they are, the fewer nutrients and more bad fats they contain	Salted, unroasted nuts—a much better alternative for satisfying hunger; one small handful, maximum	Raw, organic, unsalted nuts—protein in a clean, raw form; again, keep the quantity small—one handful only
Fried chicken—usually poor-quality meat surrounded by a layer of lard	BBQ chicken with salad—better-quality protein and a lot less fat; just take off the skin to avoid the toxins that cause cellulite (see pp. 112–14)	Turkey breast and super greens—turkey is a very lean meat that helps you sleep

Bad	Better	Best
Burger and fries—usually the bread is so sugary, it's classified as a pastry; poor-quality meat and sometimes not even real potato in the fries	Burger and salad—breadless means less empty carbs and more room for the clean salad	Lean beef stir-fry with loads of vegetables—quick and delicious; feeds your muscles and burns fat
Deep-fried fish—clogs up your heart and causes cellulite (see pp. 112–14)	Pan-fried fish and salad—if you're in a restaurant always ask for your fish to be pan fried or, better still, grilled	Grilled fish and a green salad—if you want to get rid of your cellulite, have this every night; it's the most perfect meal there is
Lamb korma (swimming in cream)	Lamb stew	Stir-fried lamb with vegetables
Pizza	Homemade pizza	Vegetable stir-fry
Sausage rolls—poor-quality meat wrapped in buttery pastry	Lamb or chicken kebab with salad	Lamb or chicken with salad
Sausage	Organic sausage	Organic steak
Battery egg	Free-range egg—one battery egg contains 15 to 30 times more cholesterol than a free-range egg; this is how eggs got their bad reputation	Organic eggs—the highest bio-availability of any protein; the gold standard!
Scrambled or fried eggs	Poached or boiled eggs	Organic or free-range poached or boiled eggs
Canned meat	Fresh meat	Fresh organic meat
Battered or crumbed fish	Fresh farmed fish	Wild/organic fish
Packaged sliced ham	Ham off the bone	Organic ham off the bone
Processed cheese slices	Block of store-bought cheese	Organic natural goat's cheese
Canned tuna	Canned mackerel	Line-caught canned sardines
Canned salmon	Farmed smoked salmon	Organic smoked salmon
Crumbed or breaded fish	Fresh fish	Wild/organic fish

Note: Omega 3 fatty acid is found in oily fish, walnuts and flaxseed. Omega 6 fatty acid is found in avocados, fish, meat, other nuts, and seeds. A good ratio for your diet is one part Omega 3 to four parts Omega 6.

Chapter 6
Your 14-day Kickstart

This chapter will reveal…

▸ Why it's worth buying organic food

▸ Why you should never microwave your food

▸ 14 days' worth of easy-to-prepare meals

This plan is flexible, in that you can add extra green vegetables to a meal if you're still hungry, and feel free to mix and match the days. For example, something like grilled sea bass is easier to cook for lunch at the weekend, rather than during the week, if you work in an office. For that reason, it's best to start the plan at the weekend when you'll have more time to prepare the meals. You'll need recipes for some of the meals (for these and more Clean & Lean recipes, see Chapter 7). In fact, if you don't like the look of some of the suggestions here, you can always substitute meal suggestions from the recipes in Chapter 7.

Options
There are plenty of non-meat options for vegetarians in the Clean & Lean plan. Just substitute the vegetarian options accordingly.

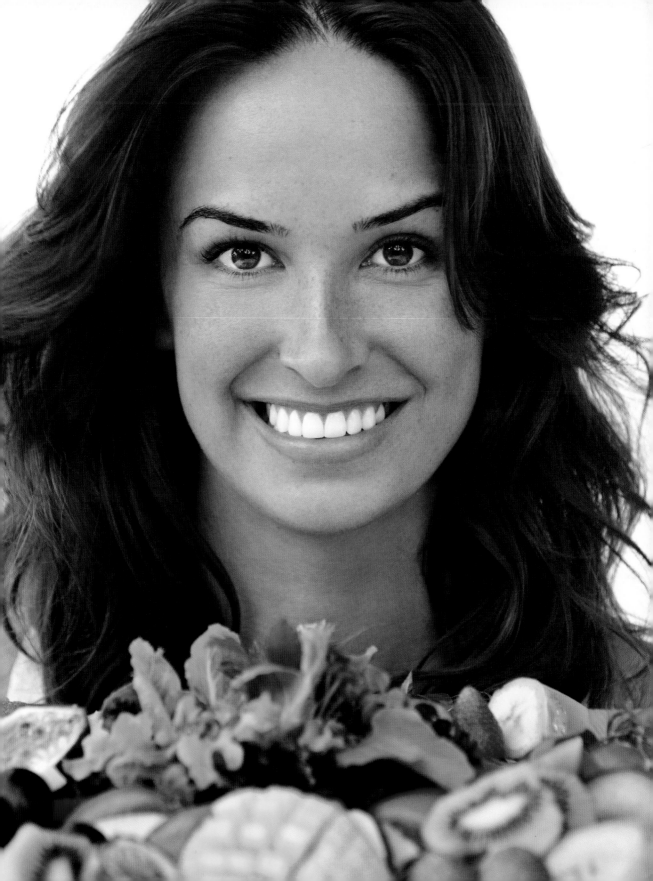

Why it's Worth Buying Organic Food

If possible, try to buy everything organic. This is especially important when it comes to vegetables, dairy, eggs, and meat.

If you do buy nonorganic chicken, always remove the skin because that's where many of the toxins are stored. And try to serve vegetables as raw as possible, and when you do cook them make sure you grill, steam, sauté, or stir-fry them, rather than frying, boiling, or microwaving.

Why You Shouldn't Microwave Your Food

The reason for this is quite simple: because it "kills" your food. If you microwave vegetables, you'll destroy most of the nutrients in them, which means your body won't be as clean as it could be. For this reason, when possible, always heat food through in a pan instead of using the microwave.

What about fruit?

My 14-day Clean & Lean Kickstart is low in fruit (although high in vegetables). This is because fruit contains so much sugar, and for this initial kickstart, I want to limit sugar intake as much as possible. Once you have done your first two weeks, you can re-introduce berries (raspberries, blueberries, strawberries). They're jam-packed with antioxidants and have a highly beneficial compound called proanthocyanidins, which protects you against degenerative diseases, such as cancer, heart disease, and diabetes. In Chapter 10 I'll talk more about reintroducing other foods and drinks after the kickstart, such as coffee and wine.

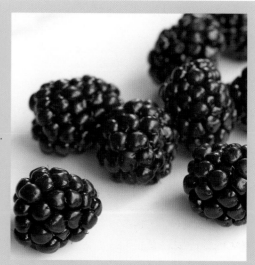

14-day Kickstart Meal Planner

Day 1

BREAKFAST: 1 boiled or scrambled egg, 2oz smoked salmon, and a cup of spinach

LUNCH: 1 grilled sea bass with a salad of mixed leaves, red peppers, green beans, broccoli, and a dash of olive oil and fresh lemon juice

SNACK: 4–6 nuts

DINNER: 3–4oz lean beef with steamed broccoli and spinach, and a quarter of an avocado

SNACK: chopped vegetables with a tablespoon of hummus

Day 2

BREAKFAST: 3–4oz smoked salmon with chopped cucumber

LUNCH: a salad made with 4oz sliced turkey, chopped tomato, cucumber, spinach leaves, quarter of an avocado with a drizzle of olive oil

SNACK: 3oz chicken with mixed raw vegetables

DINNER: 1 grilled cod fillet, served with steamed green beans/vegetables

SNACK: a small handful of seeds (try pumpkin, sunflower, etc.)

Day 3

BREAKFAST: green beans with quarter of an avocado and 3–4oz sliced chicken

LUNCH: a 2-egg omelette made with spinach and a slice of turkey, served with a green salad

SNACK: 2oz chicken

DINNER: grilled lamb chops (3–4oz) with spinach, broccoli, and red peppers

SNACK: 5 Brazil nuts

What does 3–4oz look ike?
If you don't have scales to measure out your protein portion, here's a rough guide to the measurements given in the 14-day diet plan:

▶ 3–4oz smoked salmon = the size of your outstretched hand (including fingers)
▶ 3–4oz chicken = two thirds of the size of a regular breast
▶ 3–4oz lean beef = the size of a small hamburger

Day 4

BREAKFAST: 3–4oz turkey with grilled mixed vegetables

LUNCH: a mackerel (3–4oz) salad, including tomato, baby spinach, and green beans, drizzled with olive oil

SNACK: 2oz chicken and a handful of almonds

DINNER: 1 chicken breast with steamed zucchini

SNACK: 8 cashew nuts

Day 5

BREAKFAST: 2 boiled eggs with red peppers and a quarter of an avocado

LUNCH: pan-fried shrimp (3–4oz) with sautéed mixed vegetables

SNACK: 3–4oz beef or turkey with 2 oatcakes

DINNER: 1 chicken breast, stir-fried with mixed vegetables

SNACK: 2oz chicken and a small handful of sunflower seeds

Day 6

BREAKFAST: 1 scrambled egg with spinach, cooked with extra virgin olive oil and 1 slice of turkey

LUNCH: 1 beef burger (skip the bun) with pan-fried mushrooms, onions, and grilled tomato, served with a small salad

SNACK: chopped vegetables with hummus

DINNER: baked salmon fillet (add some chopped dill, crushed garlic, and paprika to it first, wrap it in foil, and bake), served with steamed broccoli and cauliflower

SNACK: 5 Brazil nuts

Day 7

BREAKFAST: 2oz smoked salmon with a wedge of lemon and 1 poached egg

LUNCH: 3–4oz roast chicken with a large mixed salad

SNACK: 2oz sliced turkey with 2 thick slices of avocado

DINNER: 3–4oz rump steak served with peppers, green beans, and broccoli

SNACK: 4–6 nuts

Day 8

BREAKFAST: 3–4oz turkey with mixed salad

LUNCH: a 2-egg turkey and spinach omelette, served with mixed greens

SNACK: chopped vegetables with 1 tablespoon of hummus

DINNER: grilled salmon steak with sautéed kale, cabbage, and red peppers

SNACK: 4–6 macadamia nuts

Day 9

BREAKFAST: 3–4oz mackerel and half a slice of rye bread

LUNCH: baked sea bass with a salad, including tomato, baby spinach, cucumber, olives, and green beans, drizzled with olive oil

SNACK: 2oz turkey with 4–6 almonds

DINNER: 1 grilled chicken breast, served on a bed of steamed asparagus and zucchini

SNACK: 4–6 nuts

Day 10

BREAKFAST: smoked trout with carrots and red and yellow peppers

LUNCH: pan-fried shrimp (3–4oz) and spinach with fresh cilantro

SNACK: 2oz chicken with chopped vegetables

DINNER: chicken pesto (see p. 82, for recipe)

SNACK: 2oz turkey with a small handful of sunflower seeds

Day 11

BREAKFAST: 2oz turkey, 1 boiled egg, with chopped red peppers

LUNCH: 3–4oz lean beef steak, served with steamed broccoli and green beans

SNACK: 4–6 nuts

DINNER: 1 grilled chicken breast, served with green peas

SNACK: half an avocado and 2oz turkey

Day 12

BREAKFAST: 2 poached eggs with 2 grilled tomatoes

LUNCH: 1 grilled cod fillet with arugula, red onion, and snow peas

SNACK: celery, 1 tablespoon of hummus, and 1oz chicken

DINNER: 3–4oz roast turkey served with roasted peppers and broccoli

SNACK: 4–6 cashew nuts

Day 13

BREAKFAST: 2oz smoked salmon with a wedge of lemon and 1 poached egg

LUNCH: 1 grilled chicken breast with steamed vegetables or a mixed salad

SNACK: 2oz turkey with 2 thick slices of avocado

DINNER: 1 lean beef steak (3–4oz) cooked with pepper and garlic, served with steamed green beans and broccoli

SNACK: 4–6 nuts

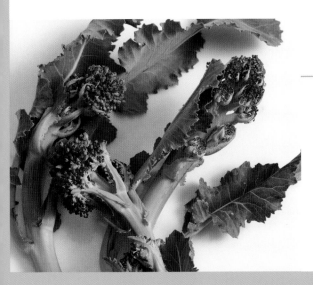

Day 14

BREAKFAST: 3–4oz smoked salmon with chopped cucumber

LUNCH: 3–4oz sliced turkey, a quarter of an avocado, and sliced tomatoes, drizzled with olive oil

SNACK: 3oz chicken with mixed raw vegetables

DINNER: 1 baked salmon steak, served with steamed mixed vegetables

SNACK: 4–6 nuts

Chapter 7
Recipes and Kitchen Must-haves

This chapter will reveal…

▸ How easy it is to make healthy meals

▸ The foods you should always have in your kitchen

▸ The smoothie that blasts fat

Food writer Nina Harris, whose love of food helped in her weight-loss success, has provided many of the recipes in this chapter. All are nutritious, fat-busting, taste great, and are easy to make.

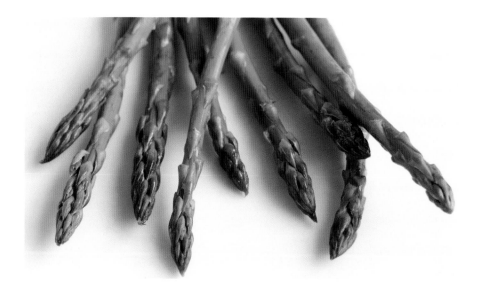

Clean & Lean Proteins

- Chicken
- Turkey
- Lamb
- Beef
- Duck
- Liver
- Pork
  (maximum once a week)
- All fish and shellfish
  (to avoid mercury, no more than two or three servings of tuna and swordfish a week)

Clean & Lean Vegetables

- Broccoli
- Spinach
- Asparagus
- Green beans
- Snow peas
- Kale
- Arugula
- Watercress
- Brussels sprouts
- Cucumber
- Zucchini
- Avocado

Clean & Lean Flavors

- Extra-virgin olive oil
  (the best you can buy)
- Walnut oil
- White wine vinegar
- Sesame oil
- Light olive oil
  (for cooking)
- Basil-infused oil
- Garlic-infused olive oil
- Flaxseed oil
- Canola oil
- Tamari soy sauce
  (gluten free)
- Good quality mayonnaise
  (keep refrigerated)
- Dijon mustard
- Lemons
- Limes
- Cilantro
- Dill
- Parsley
- Thyme
- Chile
- Cinnamon
- Garlic
- Ginger

Clean & Lean Nuts and Seeds

- Almonds
- Pecans
- Walnuts
- Brazil nuts
- Pistachios
- Macadamia nuts
- Cashews
- Chestnuts
- Sesame seeds
- Peanuts
- Sunflower seeds
- Pumpkin seeds
- Flax seed
  (ground only)

Here are my particular favorites that deserve a special mention...

Cinnamon First of all, cinnamon's most amazing property is that it can reduce blood-sugar levels (therefore hunger and cravings) and bad cholesterol. It's also an anti-inflammatory so it can help with aches and pains. Don't bother spending a fortune on cinnamon—the cheap stuff is as good as the expensive stuff. I sprinkle it in my coffee.

Garlic This helps with so many things, the list is almost too long. But here's a start: it's antiviral, an antioxidant, and helps lower bad cholesterol. Garlic is also a great tool for weight loss. The most effective way to eat it is by crushing it—the more finely crushed the better as it releases two fat-burning enzymes. So get into garlic!

Ginger This is a great antioxidant. It's also been shown to boost the immune system, help blood circulation, and aid digestion. I love having it chopped up in hot water with a slice of lemon.

Parsley I love this. It's a famous detoxifier because it will purify your body and freshen your breath. It's also used to reduce blood glucose and it has even been suggested that it is a cancer fighter.

Rosemary This is great for your brain and is used by aromatherapists the world over to improve your mood.

Sage This is another purifier, antioxidant, and anti-inflammatory. It's also good for indigestion and a sore throat. NOTE: Don't eat sage during pregnancy.

Turmeric This is used extensively in Eastern healing methods. It's an incredible anti-inflammatory and can be used for muscle and joint pain. It's also a very powerful antioxidant and great for your liver.

Breakfasts

All serve 1 (except where stated)

Bodyism Pancakes

SERVES 2–4
½ cup rolled oats
1⅓ cups fat-free cottage
   cheese
4 eggs
1 teaspoon cinnamon

Blend the ingredients in a food processor. Pour into a heated pan by the $^{1}/_{4}$ cup, cooking 2–3 minutes per side. Serve with your favorite berries.

Boiled Eggs with Spelt Bread

2 eggs
a slice of spelt bread
   (see below)

Boil the eggs and serve with a slice of the spelt bread.

Top tip! Spread olive oil on the spelt bread

How to make spelt bread

More digestible than wheat and richer in nutrients, spelt bread is fast becoming the superfood of breads with a huge celebrity following. Look out for it in supermarkets and health-food stores, or try this easy 3-minute recipe (all ingredients can be found, again, in supermarkets and health-food stores)...

4 cups spelt flour
10g fast-acting dried yeast
½ teaspoon sea salt
⅓ cup sunflower seeds
⅓ cup sesame seeds
⅓ cup flax seed
2 cups warm water

▸ Heat the oven to 400°F.
▸ Mix all the ingredients in a large bowl, adding the water last. Mix well (but don't knead it like you would while making traditional bread) until it has a doughlike consistency
▸ Put it into a greased loaf pan
▸ Bake in the oven for an hour
▸ Remove the loaf from the oven, take it out of the pan, and then return it to the oven without the pan for a further 5–10 minutes.

Omelettes

Omelettes are a fantastically healthy breakfast, since they're cheap to make and take literally minutes. It's a great idea to keep varying the fillings so you don't get bored. Follow the basic cooking method (below), then fill them up with any of the following:

2 eggs

a pinch of sea salt

a pinch of black pepper

1 teaspoon olive oil

• Turkey, mushrooms, scallions
• Fresh or dried chiles, with onions
• Zucchini and tomatoes (remove the seeds, otherwise your omelette will turn red!)
• Red bell pepper, ham, and red onion
• Smoked salmon and watercress
• Tomato, spinach, mushrooms, and basil

1 Crack the eggs into a bowl and beat with a fork until smooth. Season the eggs with salt and pepper and stir in any herbs you would like to use.

2 Heat the oil in a nonstick frying pan. When the oil is hot, add the chosen ingredients to the pan (however, if you're having tomatoes only add them at the last minute).

3 Add the egg mixture. Using a spatula and working in a circular motion, move the eggs around in the pan, while at the same time tilting the pan back and forth across the heat. Cook until golden brown underneath, but slightly soft and clear on the top. Fold the omelette over (and in half) and cook for another minute. Serve immediately.

Top tips!

▶ Chop the fillings up and store them in the fridge overnight if you're short on time.

▶ Add some chopped herbs to the egg mix to add great flavor. Try dill, basil, cilantro or parsley.

The Egg Stack

1–2 eggs
4 mushrooms, sliced
2 scallions, sliced
2oz ham
1 plum tomato, sliced

1 Poach the eggs. Alternatively, you could fry them in a nonstick pan with a tiny bit of olive oil (put the lid on the frying pan and the yolks will cook perfectly).

2 Pan-fry the mushrooms and scallions until soft and slightly brown. Gently heat the ham in the pan to warm through.

3 Arrange the ham, mushrooms, scallions, and tomato in a stack and place the poached (or fried) eggs on top.

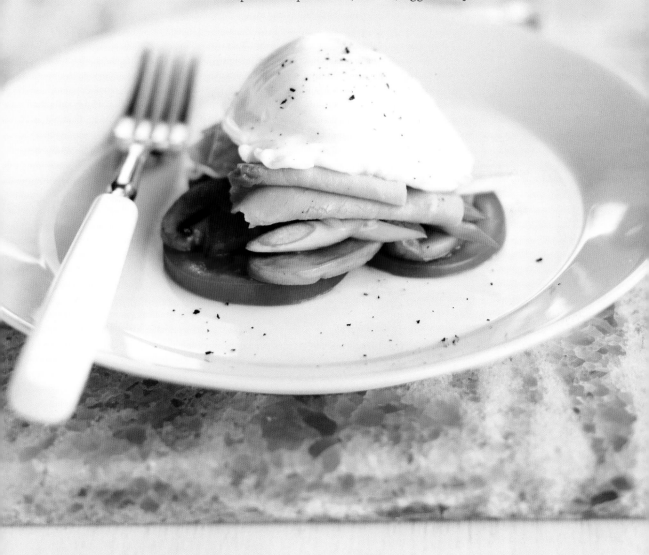

Bodyism Super Breakfast

2 tablespoons oats

2 Brazil nuts

2 almonds

2 walnuts

1 teaspoon flaxseed (ground)

1 tablespoon pumpkin seeds

1 teaspoon chia seeds

Soak the ingredients overnight in the refrigerator in a glass of rice milk and water (or cow's milk if you're able to digest it). Drink first thing—this is bursting with nutrients and goodness with a perfect balance of carbohydrates, fats, and protein, and it's particularly good for your digestion.

The Super Skinny Smoothie

2 Brazil nuts

2 almonds

a handful of blueberries and
   raspberries (around 10)

a scoop of Body Brilliance
   (see page 158)

a scoop of Body Fiber
   Ultimate Clean (see
   page 158)

a glass of water/milk/rice
   milk/almond milk

Mix all the ingredients in a blender, serve in a tall glass, and drink immediately.

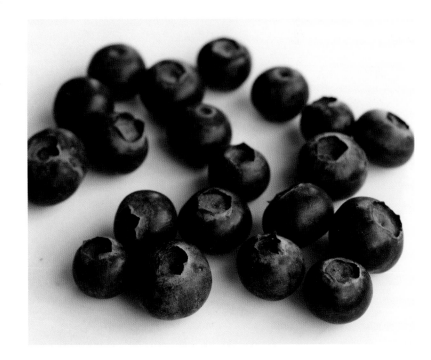

Lunches & Dinners

All serve 1 (except where stated)

Chicken stir-fry

This recipe works with any protein or vegetable combination.

1 tablespoon coconut oil

1 clove garlic, chopped

ginger, cut into long slivers (amount to taste)

1/2–1 chile, chopped (seeded if you don't like it very spicy)

1 onion, white or red, chopped

3–4oz chicken breast, sliced

asparagus

broccoli

snow peas

1 tablespoon tamari (gluten-free) soy sauce

a handful of cilantro, chopped

Heat the oil in a wok or frying pan until hot. Add the garlic, ginger, chile, and onion, and fry for 1 minute. Add the chicken and cook for about three minutes, until almost cooked through. Add the vegetables and cook for a couple of minutes, then add the soy sauce. At the last minute, stir in the cilantro.

Top tip!

▶ If you use flavorsome ingredients like fresh chile and ginger you won't need the salty, sugary sauces often used in stir-fries.

Grilled Chicken Salad

SERVES 4

1 head Romaine lettuce

1lb button mushrooms, sliced

2 cloves garlic, chopped

1 red onion, sliced

⅓ cup Parmesan cheese

½ teaspoon cracked black
pepper

4 boneless, skinless chicken
breasts

½ teaspoon sea salt

1 teaspoon chopped rosemary

1 lime

1 Tear the Romaine lettuce into bite-size pieces, and toss with the mushrooms, garlic, onion, and some olive oil. Place on chilled salad plates. Spoon 1 teaspoon of Parmesan cheese over each serving and top with cracked black pepper.

2 Season the chicken breasts with salt, pepper, and rosemary and grill for about 6 minutes per side. Slice and serve over the salad. Garnish with the remaining cheese, squeeze lime juice all over each salad, and serve immediately.

Chicken Pesto

SERVES 2

2 boneless, skinless chicken
breasts

4 teaspoons pesto

crushed black pepper

1 Preheat the oven to 375°F.

2 With a sharp knife, slice each chicken breast in half so it unfolds. Spread a teaspoon of pesto into each, then close them back up. Season the chicken with black pepper, and bake in a preheated oven for 25 minutes. Serve with a green salad.

Chicken Cajun Salad

This is quick and easy to make, and the Cajun spices add a good punch to the salad.

3–4oz boneless, skinless
  chicken breast
1 tablespoon olive oil
1–2 teaspoons Cajun spice
  mix (depending on how
  spicy you like it)
salad leaves
cucumber, sliced thinly
celery, sliced thinly
tomatoes (the best you
  can buy)
1 avocado

For the dressing:
1 tablespoon olive oil
juice of ½ lemon
1 tablespoon chopped
  cilantro (optional)

1 Cut through the middle of the chicken breast to halve the thickness of it. Rub it with olive oil and the Cajun spice mix.

2 Heat a grill pan (or other frying pan) until hot. Add the chicken and cook for several minutes on each side until cooked through.

3 Remove from the heat, and slice into strips.

4 Assemble the salad ingredients in a salad bowl. Add the dressing to the salad and toss. Serve on plates and top with chicken slices.

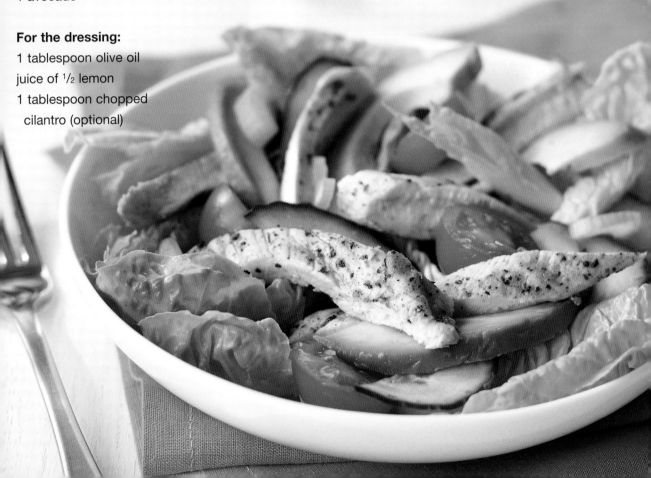

Grilled Lamb with Asparagus and Radish Salad

This one takes a while, but it's worth it—it's literally an explosion of flavor on a plate. This recipe is particularly good for the grill.

SERVES 2

2 lamb steaks (3–4oz each)

5oz asparagus

lettuce, arugula or spinach

1 tablespoon chopped mint

1 tablespoon chopped
  cilantro

½ small red onion, finely sliced

5–6 radishes, finely sliced

For the marinade:

1 tablespoon olive oil

1 chile, seeds removed, finely
  chopped

1 clove garlic, finely chopped

1 tablespoon chopped
  cilantro

1 tablespoon chopped mint

1 tablespoon chopped
  rosemary

zest of ½ lemon

a pinch of sea salt and
  black pepper

juice of ½ lemon

1 First, marinate the lamb. Combine the marinade ingredients in a bowl and mix. Add the lamb steaks and ensure they're both well covered with the marinade. Cover the dish with plastic wrap and marinate in the fridge for several hours to intensify the flavor. If you're really short of time, half an hour will be fine.

2 Next, prepare the salad. Steam or boil the asparagus for a few minutes (but ensure they remain firm and crunchy, too). Cool in ice water to ensure they don't continue cooking. Slice on the diagonal into ½ inch pieces. Add asparagus to the salad leaves, with the mint, cilantro, and the finely sliced red onion and radishes.

3 In a dry, hot grill pan, cook the lamb steaks for 2–3 minutes per side, depending on the thickness and how you like it. Three minutes a side will ensure your lamb is medium-cooked after resting. Wrap the cooked lamb in some aluminum foil for at least 5 minutes to let it rest.

4 Slice the lamb. Dress the salad with some olive oil and lemon juice. Serve the salad with the lamb slices placed on top.

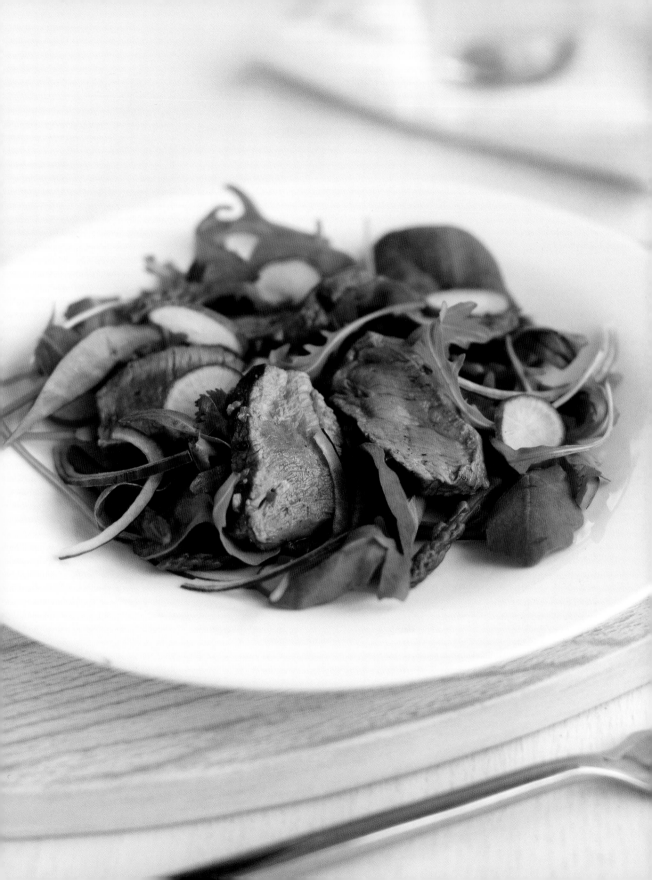

Hearty Sausage Stew

A wonderfully warming winter supper suitable for the whole family.
It also freezes well.

SERVES 4

4 red bell peppers

2 red onions

8 cloves of garlic, crushed

5 sprigs of thyme

8 large gluten-free sausages

1 x 14oz can tomatoes

a small bunch of parsley or
 cilantro

green beans

broccoli

1 Preheat the oven to 350°F. Deseed and slice the red peppers into long wide strips. Cut the onions into thin wedges. Place both in a casserole dish with the garlic cloves, thyme, and a tablespoon of olive oil. Toss, and bake in the oven for 15 minutes, or until almost soft.

2 Meanwhile, brown the sausages in a frying pan for 5–10 minutes. Add the sausages and the tomatoes to the casserole and cook for a further 30 minutes or so, until they are cooked through. Once out of the oven, sprinkle the dish with either chopped parsley or cilantro to add some extra flavor. Serve with the green beans and broccoli.

Remember! Nonorganic meat is likely to be packed with hormones that make you fat.

Umbrian Veal Chops

SERVES 2

2 veal chops

1 lemon (optional)

arugula

For the marinade:

1 handful of sage

2 large sprigs of rosemary

2 tablespoons olive oil

sea salt and black pepper

Tomato & Basil Salad

3 large tomatoes, diced

1 large handful of basil, chopped

1 tablespoon olive oil

sea salt and black pepper

1 First make the marinade. You can either finely chop the herbs and combine with the oil, salt, and pepper, or put it all in a mini food processor and blitz it. Cover the chops in the marinade and, if possible, leave in fridge for several hours. Make the tomato and basil salad by combining all the ingredients. This is even better if you make it half an hour before serving as it allows the flavor of the basil to penetrate the tomatoes.

2 Pan-fry the chops in a hot nonstick pan for about 5 minutes a side, depending on thickness. Ensure you take them off the heat when they seem to be medium-rare because they will continue to cook when off the heat. Let them rest for 5 minutes, by which time they will be nice and juicy. Add a squeeze of lemon juice and serve with the basil salad and some arugula on the side.

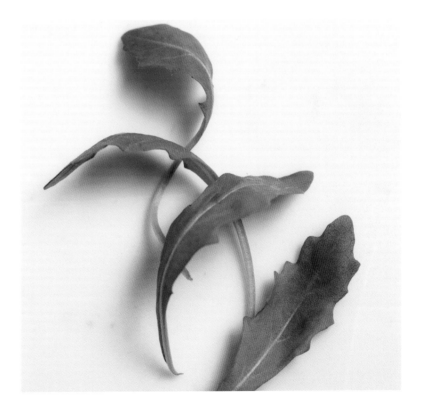

Simple Bouillabaisse

The ultimate one-pot, simple seafood dinner. Use any combination of seafood you like. For some extra zing add the rind of half an orange.

SERVES 2

1 tablespoon olive oil

1 small onion, diced

1 clove garlic, finely chopped

1 medium fennel bulb, diced

2 bay leaves

2 cups fish stock

a pinch of saffron

¾ cup chopped tomatoes

a small handful of parsley (to serve)

Mixed seafood:

1 white fish fillet (8oz), cut into large chunks

8oz mussels (in shells)

2oz shrimp

For the rouille (optional):

1 tablespoon mayonnaise

½ clove garlic, finely chopped

¼ teaspoon cayenne pepper

a pinch of saffron

1 First make the rouille. Mix all the ingredients in a bowl and set aside.

2 Prepare the seafood. Cut up the fish into large chunks. Clean the mussels and lightly tap them—they should close. If not, discard them. Peel and devein the shrimp.

3 In a large cast-iron pot (with a lid), cook the diced onion in the olive oil for 2 minutes on a medium heat. The idea is to cook lightly the vegetables. Add the garlic, fennel, and bay leaves and cook for a further 2 minutes. Turn up the heat, pour in the stock, saffron, and tomatoes. Once bubbling, add the seafood and cook until the fish is cooked through and the mussels have opened (about 4–5 minutes).

4 Spoon the seafood and the lovely fragrant broth and vegetables in bowls and sprinkle with parsley. Add a small spoonful of the rouille if you wish.

Salmon Fillet with Dill Salad

sugar snap peas*
snow peas*
½ small red onion*, diced
1 tablespoon chopped dill
1 tablespoon extra-virgin
 olive oil
juice of ½ lemon
sea salt and black pepper
1 salmon fillet (3–4oz)

*You can have as much or as little of these as you like, and can even leave one or two out and replace with another vegetable if you don't like them.

1 First, prepare the salad. In a medium saucepan, bring some water to a boil. When it's boiling, add a generous pinch of salt and the sugar snap peas. After 20 seconds of boiling, add the snow peas. Keep on the heat for a further 20 seconds, then drain, and run under cold water. Even better is to plunge the vegetables into a bowl of iced water. This will stop them cooking in their tracks! You want them to stay crunchy but blanching them in the boiling water brings out their flavor.

2 Dry the vegetables and place them in a bowl. Add the red onions, chopped dill, olive oil and lemon juice, and some salt and pepper.

3 Meanwhile, rub olive oil, salt and pepper on the salmon fillet. Heat a grill pan until hot. Cook the salmon fillet, skin side down, for a few minutes (depending on how thick the fillet is), then turn and cook for a final minute or so.

3 Serve the salmon with the dill salad on the side. Have extra lemon wedges for the salmon if needed.

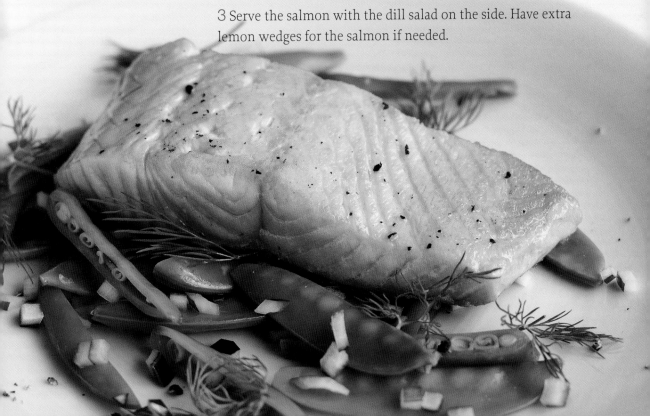

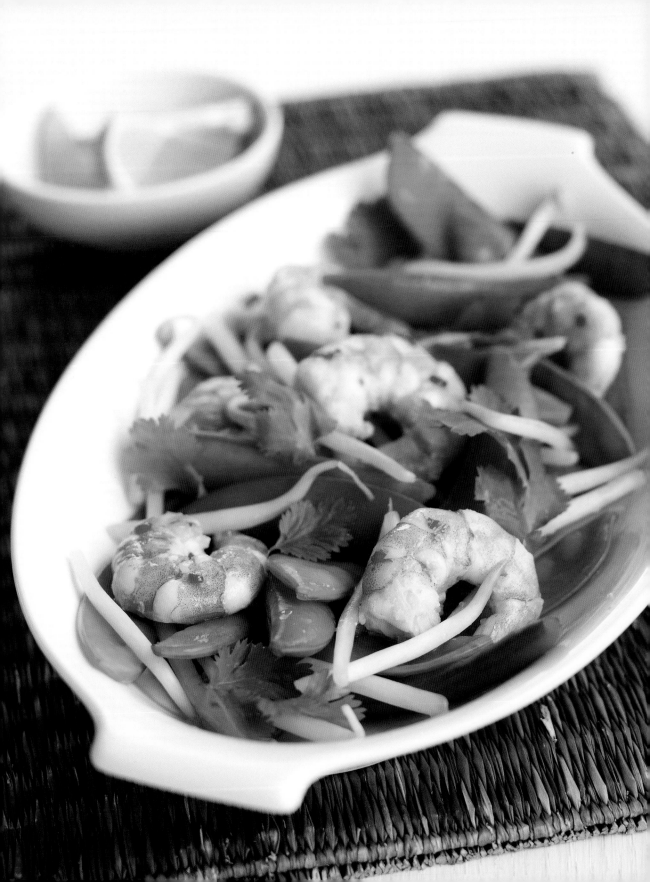

Garlic Shrimp

A different take on the 1970s classic. You can vary the recipe by serving just the shrimp with a salad.

3–4oz shrimp
a large handful of vegetables—
   good choices include
   asparagus, sugar snap peas,
   snow peas, bean sprouts,
   and chopped cilantro

For the marinade:
1 teaspoon ginger, thinly sliced
   (optional)
1 chile, seeded and finely
   diced
1 clove of garlic
small handful of parsley,
   chopped
juice of 1/2 lemon
olive oil

1 Mix the shrimp with the marinade and refrigerate, covered, for 1 hour, or just 10 minutes if you're in a hurry. You can also use frozen shrimp—they will defrost quickly in the marinade.

2 Heat a wok or frying pan. When hot, add the shrimp and stir-fry for a minute or so. As they start to turn pink, add the vegetables (except the bean sprouts) and cook for another few minutes until the shrimp are cooked. If you're using bean sprouts, add them last, along with the cilantro and a squeeze of lemon juice, and cook until heated through (it should only take a minute). Serve immediately.

Marinated Steak with Watercress

SERVES 4

4 sirloin steaks

2 large bunches of watercress

1 tablespoon extra-virgin
  olive oil

1 tablespoon walnut oil

For the marinade:

5 tablespoons tamari or soy
  sauce (gluten-free)

3 tablespoons sesame oil

3 tablespoons chopped
  cilantro

1/2–1 red chile, seeded and
  finely chopped

1 stalk lemongrass, finely
  sliced

2 tablespoons chopped ginger

2 cloves garlic, chopped

1 First, make the marinade. Combine all the marinade ingredients in a shallow dish that will fit the steaks. Coat the steaks with the marinade, cover in plastic wrap, and refrigerate for a few hours or as long as time will allow.

2 Take the steaks out of the fridge about half an hour before you wish to cook them to allow them to come to room temperature. Heat a frying pan. Remove the steaks from the marinade (leaving the rest of the marinade in the dish) and cook them in the pan. While cooking the steaks, heat the marinade in a small saucepan over low heat until warm.

3 When the steak is done to your taste, take it off the heat and let it rest in foil for several minutes. Wash the watercress and dress it with olive oil and walnut oil.

4 Cut the steak into slices, drizzle with some warm marinade, and serve alongside the watercress.

Remember! Watercress is a superfood and provides concentrated antioxidant protection.

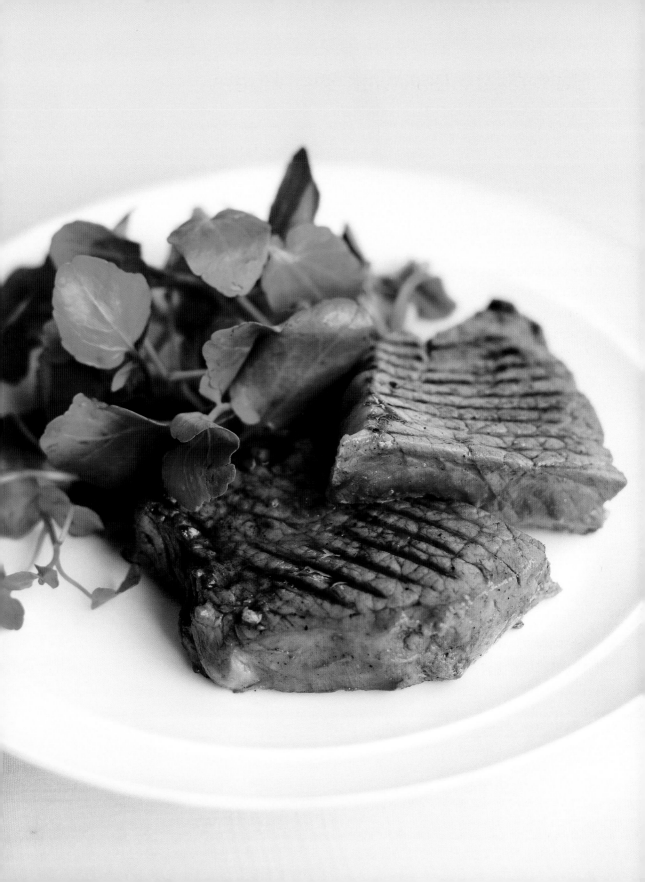

Broiled Chicken with Basil Butter

SERVES 4

4 chicken breast halves, boneless and skinless, pounded thin

3/4 teaspoon black pepper

4 tablespoons melted organic butter

a handful of basil leaves, cut into thin strips

1/2 teaspoon sea salt

For the basil butter:

3 tablespoons organic butter, at room temperature

3 tablespoons chopped basil leaves

1 tablespoon grated Parmesan cheese

1/4 teaspoon crushed garlic

1/4 teaspoon sea salt

a sprinkling of black pepper

1 In a small bowl, combine the ingredients for the basil butter and mix well. Place on a sheet of plastic wrap, form into a log, wrap tightly and refrigerate until needed.

2 Preheat the grill. Press the black pepper into the side of each chicken breast half. In a small bowl, mix the melted butter, basil, and salt. Brush each breast half with the butter mixture. Cook under the broiler, for about 7–8 minutes per side until cooked through. When the chicken is cooked, serve with the basil butter.

Bodyism Guacamole

2 medium tomatoes

2 big ripe avocadoes

1 small red onion, chopped

a little chile

1 tablespoon of lemon or lime juice

1/2 teaspoon sea salt

Remove the pulp and seeds from the tomatoes, cut into little cubes, and keep separate until just before serving. Put the flesh of the avocadoes into a bowl with the chopped onion and everything else. Add some black pepper and mash together. Add the tomato and serve immediately.

Broiled Chicken in Olive Oil and Chive Vinaigrette

SERVES 4

6 tablespoons olive oil

1 teaspoon sea salt

$1/2$ teaspoon black pepper

$1/4$ teaspoon mustard

1 clove garlic

zest of 1 lemon

1 tablespoon chopped chives

4 chicken whole breasts on
the bone, quartered

1 In a blender, process 2 tablespoons of the olive oil, $1/4$ teaspoon of the salt, pepper, and the mustard for 15 seconds. While the blender is still running, add 2 more tablespoons of the olive oil and process for 10 seconds. Add the remaining olive oil, garlic, and lemon zest. Add the chives and process for about 15 seconds more.

2 Dip each piece of chicken in the sauce, coating it well. Marinate in the fridge for at least 4 hours (or ideally overnight). Place the chicken under a preheated broiler, skin side up, about 8 inches from the heat. Sprinkle with the remaining sea salt and pepper. Grill, turning and basting with sauce every 10 minutes, for about 20 minutes or until a fork can be inserted in the chicken with ease and it is piping hot throughout.

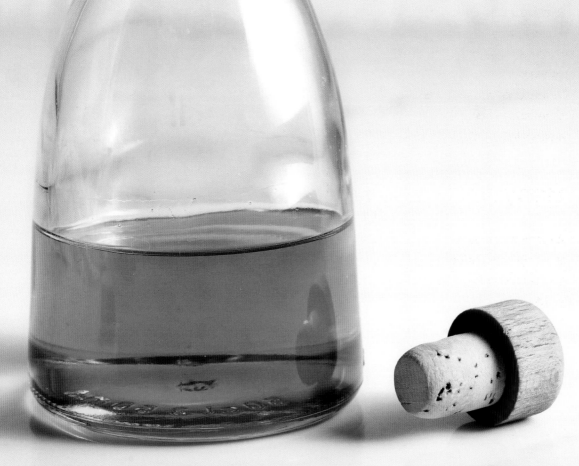

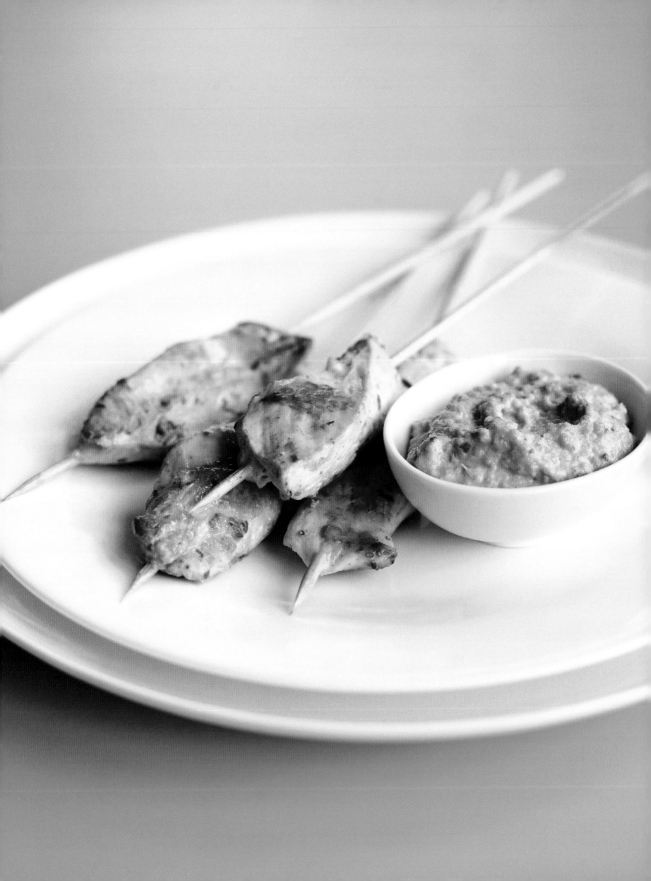

Thai Chicken Satay

MAKES 4 APPETIZERS

1 large chicken breast

2 tablespoons fish sauce

1/4 teaspoon ground cumin

1/2 cup lime juice

a good handful of cilantro

1 large clove garlic, crushed

1 stalk lemongrass, crushed

Spicy Peanut Sauce

1 tablespoon safflower oil

1/2 red onion, chopped

1 large clove garlic, crushed

1 stalk lemongrass, crushed

1/4 cup peanuts

3/4 cup low-fat coconut milk

1 teaspoon ground cumin

1 tablespoon sugar

2 tablespoons fresh lime juice

1/4 teaspoon sea salt

1 tablespoon soy sauce

1/2 teaspoon Asian hot chili oil

For the Spicy Peanut Sauce

Place the safflower oil in a small pan over a medium heat. Add the red onion, crushed garlic and lemongrass. Cook, stirring, for about 3 minutes; remove from heat. In a food processor, crush the peanuts; add the onion mixture, low-fat coconut milk, ground cumin, sugar, fresh lime or lemon juice, sea salt, oy sauce, and Asian hot chili sauce or oil. Process until smooth.

Place the chicken between sheets of wax paper and pound gently with a rolling pin to flatten slightly. Cut the chicken into diagonal strips about 1/2 inch thick. Thread a chicken strip onto 4 bamboo skewers.

In a shallow bowl, place the fish sauce, safflower oil, lime juice, cilantro, garlic, cumin, and lemongrass; stir to mix well. Dip each skewer into the mixture, turning to coat chicken. Place the chicken in a dish, cover with plastic wrap, and refrigerate for at least 2 hours or, ideally, overnight. Cook the chicken under a hot broiler, about 3–4 minutes per side or until it's no longer pink inside. Serve with the Spicy Peanut Sauce.

Garlic Lime Chicken

SERVES 4

4 chicken breast halves

1/4 cup fresh lime juice

1/4 cup Worcestershire sauce

2 cloves garlic, crushed

1/2 teaspoon mustard powder

1/2 teaspoon coarsely ground
  black pepper

Mix together the lime juice, Worcestershire sauce, garlic, and mustard. Place the chicken in a bowl and pour the sauce over it. Cover and marinate in the fridge for 30 minutes. Remove the chicken from the marinade and sprinkle with pepper. Heat up the marinade in a pan over medium heat, add the chicken, and cook for about 8 minutes on each side or until the chicken is cooked and piping hot all the way through. Serve immediately.

Note: This is delicious served hot or cold.

Super Ground Beef

The thing that's so super about this is that it's cheap, easy, and bursting with nutrition. The recipe is always evolving and should contain pretty much whatever vegetables you have in your fridge.

SERVES 4

1 red bell pepper

1 zucchini

a handful of peas

a good handful of broccoli

1 eggplant

olive oil

fresh rosemary

1lb lean organic ground beef

14oz organic tomato sauce

a pinch of parsley

a pinch of rosemary

2 cloves garlic, finely chopped

Chop all the vegetables up into nice big chunks. Brown the ground beef in a pot with a little olive oil and some fresh rosemary. Then add the chopped up vegetables and organic tomato sauce and simmer for about half an hour. Add the parsley and any extra rosemary. Stir it for a few more minutes, then right at the end add the garlic and stir through. If you want, you can serve it with a little brown rice on the side (but I prefer it without).

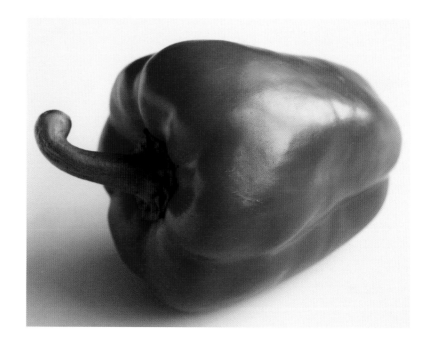

Grilled Caribbean Chicken Breasts

SERVES 4

4 boneless chicken breast
halves

1 tablespoon orange zest

1 tablespoon olive oil

1 tablespoon lime juice

1 tsp crushed fresh ginger

1/4 cup orange juice

2 cloves garlic, crushed

1/2 teaspoon Louisiana hot
sauce (you can get some
great hot sauces in most
major supermarkets—buy to
your own taste)

1/2 teaspoon fresh oregano

Place the chicken breasts in a folded piece of plastic wrap; slightly flatten the upper portion of each breast with a rolling pin. Place the breasts in a shallow glass dish. Combine the remaining ingredients in a small bowl and pour over the chicken. Cover with plastic wrap and marinate in the fridge for at least 2 hours (or up to 4). Remove the breasts from the marinade and place them under a preheated broiler and cook for about 6–8 minutes on each side.

Top of Form Bodyism Super Salad

SERVES 2

4 handfuls of baby spinach

1 cucumber, diced

1 red bell pepper, diced

2 handfuls of mung-bean
sprouts

2 handfuls of cherry tomatoes

4 tablespoons pumpkin and
sunflower seeds

a sprinkling of pine nuts

1 avocado

a drizzle of extra-virgin olive oil

Stir, mix, and enjoy.

You can vary the ingredients if you want, but remember that tomatoes are full of lycopene, which neutralizes the free radicals that cause damage to the cells in the body.

Bombay Chicken Wings

SERVES 6–8 AS AN APPETIZER

15–20 chicken wings

1 teaspoon curry powder

$^1/_2$ teaspoon ground turmeric

2 tablespoons vegetable oil

2 tablespoons finely sliced
  scallion

2 cloves garlic, crushed

a sprinkling of black pepper

sprigs of cilantro for garnish

Yogurt Chutney Dipping Sauce

$^1/_2$ cup plain yogurt

1 tablespoon chopped cilantro

1 tablespoon finely sliced
  scallion

$^1/_4$ teaspoon hot sauce

a pinch of sea salt

1 To make the dipping sauce, combine all the ingredients in a
bowl; cover and refrigerate until needed.

2 In a large bowl, mix all the ingredients (except the chicken
wings and cilantro) to make the marinade. Add the chicken,
making sure all pieces are coated well. Cover and refrigerate for
at least 1 hour. Preheat the oven to 375°F and put the chicken
wings in a baking dish. Bake for 25 minutes until golden brown.
Serve with the dipping sauce and garnish with the cilantro sprigs.

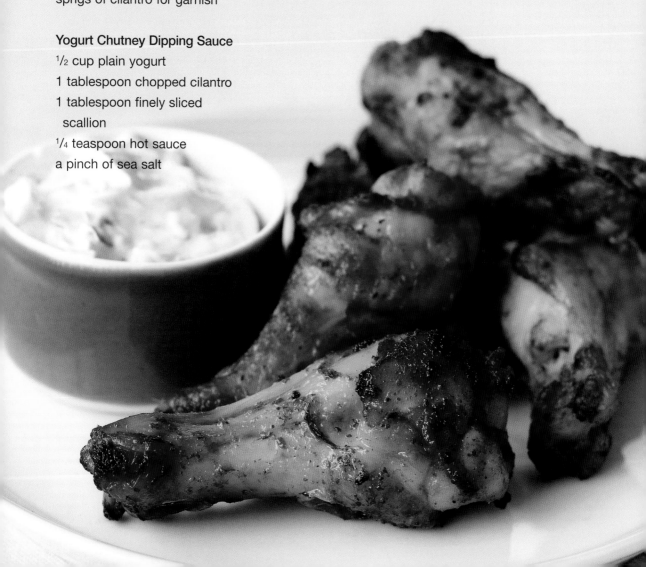

Broiled Chicken Breasts with Spicy Salsa

SERVES 4

4 boneless, skinless chicken
  breast halves

4 tablespoons fresh lime juice

¼ cup olive oil

½ teaspoon chili powder

¼ teaspoon black pepper

1 *For the Spicy Salsa*
In a bowl, mix together half a finely chopped red onion, 1 tablespoon fresh lime juice, 1 large clove garlic (crushed), 2 teaspoons seeded and finely sliced jalapeño pepper, 2 tablespoons finely chopped cilantro, ¼ teaspoon ground cumin, and ½ teaspoon sea salt. Let rest at room temperature for about 1 hour.

2 In a shallow dish, mix together the lime juice, olive oil, chili powder, and pepper. Dip the chicken in the mixture, turning to coat. Marinate in refrigerator at least 1 hour. Place chicken under a preheated broiler, skin side down, at least 7 inches from the heat. Grill for about 8 minutes either side, or until a fork can be inserted in the chicken with ease and juices run clear, not pink.

3 Remove the chicken and put on individual plates. Spoon the Spicy Salsa over each piece and garnish with avocado wedges. Sprinkle with cilantro and serve immediately.

Turkey with Asian Slaw

SERVES 2

7oz cooked turkey breast

Salad ingredients:

1 medium carrot, grated

1 small white cabbage, finely shredded

1 red pepper, finely sliced

1 large handful radishes, finely sliced into strips

For the dressing:

1 tablespoon olive oil

$1/2$ tablespoon sesame oil

2 tablespoons lime juice

3 tablespoons chopped cilantro

1 tablespoon chopped mint

1 chile, seeded and finely diced

1 First, make the dressing by combining the ingredients and mixing well.

2 Next, assemble all the vegetables in a large bowl. The trick is to slice everything as thinly as possible. Toss through the dressing. Serve with the turkey.

Top tip!

▸ Mint is great for aiding the digestion, which helps clean out the body.

Remember! Turkey is loaded with an amino acid called trytophan, which can aid sleeping.

Chicken and Cashew Stir-fry

SERVES 4

2 skinless chicken breast fillets
 ½ inch thick strips
3 tablespoons vegetable oil
2oz unsalted cashew nuts
2 cloves garlic, crushed
6 scallions, sliced
8oz broccoli, cut into bite-size
 pieces
2 long red chiles, thinly sliced
8oz snow peas, topped, tailed,
 and sliced lengthwise
⅓ cup chicken stock or water
juice of 1 lime

1 Heat a wok over a high heat. Add half the oil and, when hot, add the chicken and cashew nuts and stir-fry for 3–4 minutes or until the chicken is almost cooked through. Remove from the wok and set aside.

2 Add the remaining oil to the wok over a high heat. Add the garlic, scallions and broccoli and stir-fry for 2 minutes. Add the chiles, snow peas, and stock (or water) and stir-fry for 2 minutes or until the snow peas are bright green. Return the chicken to the wok, and stir-fry until heated through. Mix in the lime juice. Season to taste and serve with lime wedges.

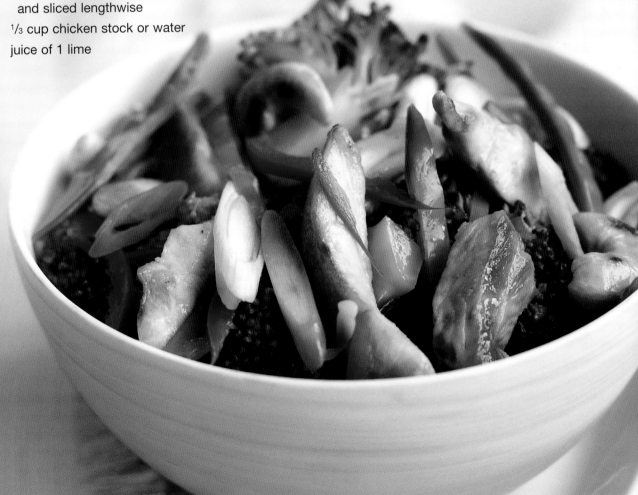

Zucchini Salad

SERVES 2

4 zucchini

1 large clove garlic

1 tablespoon olive oil

$^1/_2$–1 chile, chopped

juice of 1 lemon

2 tablespoons chopped mint

Thinly slice two zucchini lengthwise. Mix with the garlic and olive oil. Preheat a frying pan and add the zucchini, cooking on each side for about 3 minutes. Put on a serving plate, squeeze lemon juice over it, and scatter with mint and finely sliced chile. Serve with grilled chicken.

Warm Watercress and Pine Nut Salad

SERVES 2

$^1/_4$ cup olive oil

1 large clove garlic

$^1/_4$ cup pine nuts

$^1/_4$ cup hazelnuts, finely chopped

2–3 slices bacon, diced

$^1/_2$ teaspoon sea salt

$^1/_2$ teaspoon black pepper

1lb watercress, finely chopped

Gently heat the olive oil. Cut the garlic clove in half lengthwise and add it to the oil. Cook for 2 minutes, stirring constantly. Remove the garlic and discard. Add all the nuts and cook for 5–6 minutes, or until they're browned. Add the bacon, salt, and pepper. Cook for 2–3 minutes. Dry the watercress before you add it to the oil. Stir the watercress into the mixture, making sure it's well coated and barely heated through. If left too long, it loses some of its crispiness. Season with pepper and serve immediately.

Spinach Salad

SERVES 6

2 bunches fresh spinach

1 bunch scallions, chopped

juice of 1 lemon

¹/₄ tablespoon olive oil

black pepper, to taste

Wash spinach well. Drain and chop, then squeeze out the excess water. Add the scallions, lemon juice, oil, and pepper.

Remember! Organic vegetables can contain up to twice as many vitamins as nonorganic ones. And the more nutrients your body consumes, the less hungry it feels and the less it craves sugar.

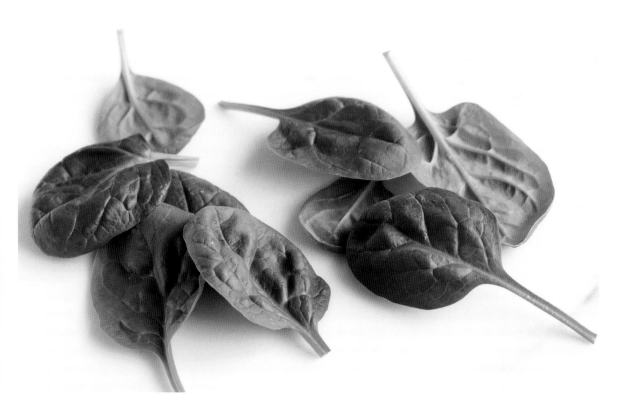

Squid with Red Onions and Kale

Kale has powerful antioxidant properties, and is anti-inflammatory.
The recipe also works well, though, with baby spinach.

SERVES 2

1 large or 2 medium squid

½ teaspoon paprika

1 clove garlic, crushed

1 tablespoon olive oil

1 lemon

a large bunch of curly kale

1 red onion

juice of ½ lemon

1 When you buy the squid, ask for it to be cleaned. Once you get it home, give it a further wash and cut it down the backbone (you can see the ridge). Cut diagonal patterns into the inside of the flesh (this will make it curl nicely when cooking). Cut into long strips.

2 Next, make the marinade: combine the paprika, garlic, olive oil, and a generous pinch of salt and pepper in a large bowl. Add the squid. You can marinate this for an hour or so, or just for 5 minutes (while you prepare the vegetables).

3 Next prepare the kale. Boil it for 3 minutes. You want to partially cook it so that it still has some bite. While this is cooking, slice the red onion, and cook with a little oil in a wok for a minute or so. Add the squid to the wok and cook on a high heat for a minute, keeping most of the marinade in the bowl. Add the kale and the remaining marinade and cook for a further 3 minutes. Squeeze the lemon juice into the pan. Remove from the heat and serve.

Sea Bass with Asparagus and Tartare Sauce

SERVES 2

2 sea bass fillets (approximately 4oz each)

a large bunch of asparagus

1 lemon

For the tartare sauce:

2 teaspoons good-quality mayonnaise

1 teaspoon baby capers, finely chopped

2 baby cornichons, finely diced

a small handful of cilantro, finely chopped

juice of ½ lemon

sea salt and black pepper

1 To make tartare sauce, mix all the ingredients together in a small bowl and set to one side.

2 Wash the sea bass and pat dry with a paper towel (you need to get rid of all the water to help the fish skin crisp up in the pan). Using your hands, rub olive oil on both sides of the sea bass fillets. Season with salt and pepper on both sides. Set to one side.

3 Steam the asparagus.

4 Heat a nonstick pan until it is hot. Add the sea bass, skin side down, and cook for a few minutes until most of the flesh appears cooked. Turn and cook for another minute or so.

5 Serve the fish and asparagus immediately, squeezing lemon juice over both. Serve the tartare sauce on the side.

Remember! The more fresh flavors you put in your food, the better it will taste and the easier it will be to avoid all those nasty artificial flavors associated with processed sugar and additives.

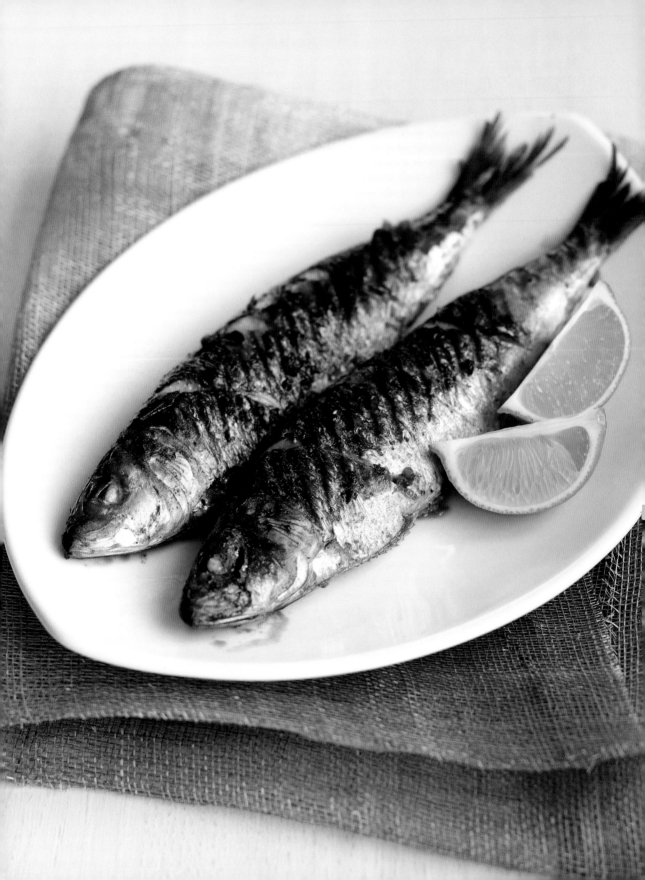

Sublime Sardines

We all need to try to eat more oily fish, but for some the strong flavor can make it difficult. This recipe should help change that.

SERVES 2
8 sardines, whole, gutted
1 clove garlic
1 tablespoon baby capers
2 tablespoons sunblushed
  tomatoes
zest of 1 lemon
2 sprigs of thyme
2 tablespoons olive oil
sea salt and black pepper

1 Get your local fish store to gut and clean the sardines.

2 Make the marinade by combining all the ingredients except the sardines in a small food processor; blend to form a rough paste. Alternatively, chop the ingredients up and mix and mash together.

3 Wash and dry the sardines and make 3 diagonal slits on each side of the body. Rub the marinade all over the fish and into the slits. Marinate for a few hours if you can; at least half an hour if you're short of time.

4 Place sardines under a hot broiler or on a grill for a few minutes each side until cooked through. Serve with steamed green beans or spinach. These are also fabulous with a salad dressed with extra-virgin olive oil and lemon juice.

Top tip!
▶ Sardines are packed with omega 3 fatty acids, which are great for your waistline, skin, and energy levels.

Chapter 8
Detox Yourself Beautiful

This chapter will reveal...

▸ Beauty tricks to help you slim down and look younger

▸ The bath that can help you lose weight

▸ How Clean & Lean gets rid of cellulite

The Clean & Lean diet is all about helping your body to shed toxins as effortlessly as possible. This chapter will focus on how detoxing can make you look, as well as feel, better.

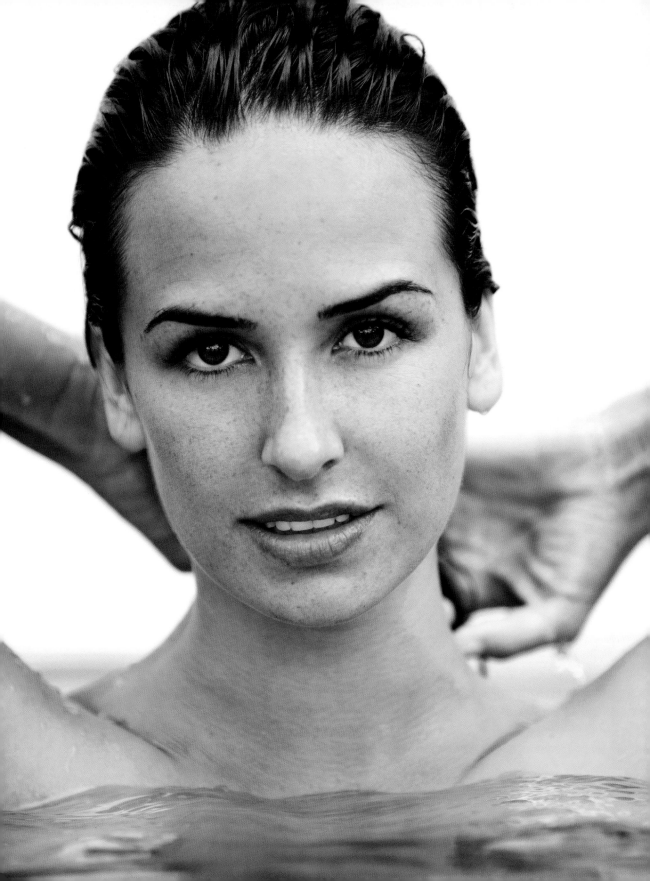

Clean & Lean Beauty

Much has been made of the chemicals in beauty products and, while the jury is still out, during the 14-day Kickstart it might be worth switching to organic beauty products. Some studies out there suggest that some of the chemicals in nonorganic beauty products end up in your system, though only small amounts—and there's no suggestion as yet that they do any real harm. But as you're detoxing your system anyway, anything that limits the amount of toxins in your body can't be a bad thing (plus lots of the most exclusive, A-list spas worldwide use organic beauty during their detox regimes).

You don't have to replace your entire bathroom cabinet and makeup bag either, just buy whatever you can afford. If you've given up your frequent trips to the pricey coffee shops and that midafternoon muffin (which you should have done by now!), then you'll have saved yourself some money to pay for it. The best products to replace are the ones that touch (and therefore sink into) your skin the most—and the ones that you don't wash off. For example, face cream, body lotion, and foundation soak in more because they cover a wider area of skin and because you need to use more of them. So if you can afford it, replace these products rather than those that touch your skin least and you wash off, such as shampoo, conditioner, mascara, eye shadow, and lipstick. There are so many fantastic organic beauty ranges out there—go for Organic Pharmacy (www.theorganicpharmacy.com), Liz Earle (us.lizearle.com), and Tisserand (www.tisserand.com).

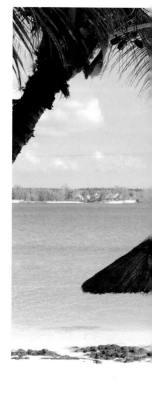

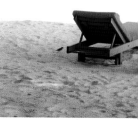

Beauty Tricks to Help You Slim Down and Look Younger

Why sugar can make you look old

In Chapter 2 we looked at how sugar can make you fat and ill. But sugar is also potentially one of the biggest aging culprits there is, as it can speed up the appearance of fine lines and wrinkles. When your blood-sugar levels rise, sugar attaches itself to the collagen fibers in your skin. Collagen is the "building brick" of the skin, helping it to stay firm, plump, and youthful

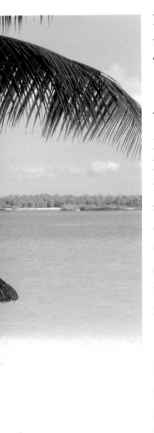

looking. When collagen breaks down (usually with age), your skin begins to appear old, wrinkled, and sagging. Too much sugar can break down this "building brick" prematurely, and makes skin less plump and elastic.

The Bath That Will Help You to Lose Weight

For a truly lazy way to ditch the toxins, try taking an Epsom salt bath. Elle—and many of my other model clients—swears by this trick. If a client is getting ready for a photo shoot or a vacation, I tell them to soak in Epsom salts in the days leading up to it—the salts are full of magnesium and encourage the body to shed toxins quickly (and remember, these toxins encourage water retention and cling on to fat). The salts also boost your digestion and reduce cellulite. Pour two cupfuls into a hot bath and soak in it for at least 20 minutes up to three times a week. Epsom salts are available from pharmacies and health-food stores.

How Clean & Lean Gets Rid of Cellulite

Cellulite is a toxic fat that has pushed its way up through the deeper layers of the skin, creating the textured (or "orange peel") appearance on the skin. It's found mainly in fatty areas, like the thighs, bottom, and stomach, but it can also be found on the upper arms.

The more toxic your system is from environmental and dietary pollutants, the more prone to cellulite you'll be. Smoking and living in a busy city toxify your body and encourage dimply thighs. But the worst cellulite

The 1-minute body trick to get rid of cellulite

Every single morning, dry-body brush yourself all over. Using a decent body brush (they're available in supermarkets and pharmacies), brush yourself before your shower or bath (not during or after, when your skin will be wet). Start at your feet and brush in light sweeps in the direction of your heart. Go easy on the softer parts of your skin, such as your tummy or breasts. This is quick, cheap, and it'll speed up the whole Clean & Lean process, get your blood pumping, and help to reduce the appearance of cellulite. Buy a brush today and get into the habit!

offenders are sugar, alcohol, and CRAP (caffeine, refined sugar, alcohol, and processed foods – see Chapter 3).

What to avoid

The wrong type of water

Yes, really. Tap water can be full of hormones, chemicals, and additives, and is the worst type for cellulite. Instead, drink filtered or bottled water, ideally from glass bottles. The more pure the water, the less prone to cellulite you will be. Aim for at least 10 cups a day.

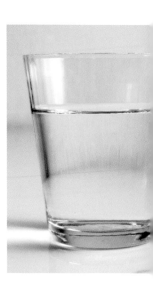

A toxic environment

As we know, city living causes cellulite. Smog, fumes, and smoking all accumulate and add stress to your body. Avoid these environments whenever possible and try to exercise in nature and away from pollution: for example, walk in the park, not along the road.

Alcohol

Regularly drinking alcohol is a major contributor to cellulite. It's the first thing that needs to go (or at least to be cut back), if you're serious about getting rid of your cellulite.

Poor circulation

Spending too many hours sitting at a desk isn't good for circulation or burning body fat. Try and get up and stretch, walk around, and sneak in some full squats (if you can) every hour or so (see p. 129).

What to do

Eat organically

Try to make sure all your food is organic as it means zero chemicals to toxify your body. This is particularly important when it comes to meat, fish, and dairy.

Cut back on coffee

Caffeine makes cellulite worse. Your everyday coffee is a contributor to slowing down your detoxification pathways including your liver (the main organ responsible for detoxing and burning fat). One a day is fine, but any more and you'll increase your chances of getting cellulite.

Ditch the refined carbs

Eating potato chips, fries, breads, and wheat-based breakfast cereals not only adds loads of calories to your diet, but also contributes to cellulite because of the bad fats these foods contain.

Eat antioxidant-rich fruits

Dark berries (such as blueberries, blackberries, and raspberries) all contain high amounts of antioxidants. Also, if you can get your hands on it, the "acai" berry from Brazil contains a higher level of antioxidants than any other known food and is a great cellulite blitzer. I put a teaspoon of freeze-dried acai in my smoothie every morning.

Drink green tea

Green tea contains massive amounts of antioxidants. It's also an excellent alternative to coffee and it helps detox your whole body.

Exercise

Regular exercise helps to promote blood flow and increase your lean muscle mass. The more lean muscle mass you have, the less fat/cellulite you will have!

Clean & Lean Around the Home

What applies to your beauty routine also applies to your household cleaning products—there are no firm studies saying that the chemicals in regular bleach, polish, or surface cleaners do any harm, but why not go for a slightly less toxic version? Especially during the 14-day Kickstart.

Again, it's about being practical and only swapping what you can afford. Madonna and Gwyneth Paltrow—and lots of other A-listers—use Method cleaning products (well, I imagine they have cleaners that use them but you get my drift!). Method is a brilliant range of chemical-free products using lots of lovely, clean ingredients such as pink grapefruit and fresh lavender. They don't cost much more than regular products, they're very eco-friendly, and you don't even have to wear rubber gloves while using them because they're so natural and toxin-free (www.methodhome.com).

Bad	Better	Best
Beer—this is packed with sugar, yeast, and alcohol; bad news for cellulite	Half juice, half water—if you're serious about getting rid of your cellulite, alcohol is the first thing that must go	Water—it flushes your kidneys, liver and cellulite; drink at least 10 cups of filtered water a day
Instant coffee—highly processed and full of toxins that clog your liver; also robs your body of nutrients	Peppermint tea—caffeine-free and an excellent digestive aid	Hot water with 2 or 3 slices of lemon and fresh ginger—this tonic has a cleansing effect on the liver, which helps banish cellulite
White bread—contains very little fiber and protein, the two nutrients that fill you up	Rye bread—a wheat-free grain that has loads of fiber	Super Salad (see p. 99 for the recipe)—all those greens are a great cellulite-zapper
Soft drinks—packed with sugar, caffeine, and empty calories	Freshly squeezed fruit juice—all natural sugars with some nutritional value	A super juice mainly made from greens—accelerates fat loss and helps cellulite: mix watercress, parsley, spinach, zucchini, green peppers, and ginger and drink immediately
Alcopop—contains both alcohol and high amounts of sugar: two ingredients that guarantee cellulite	Vodka with mineral water and a squeeze of lime—clean spirit with far fewer calories	Mineral water with a squeeze of fresh lime—if you're serious about cellulite then this is the only drink
Potato chips—the thinner the chip is, the fewer nutrients and more bad fats it contains	Salted, unroasted nuts—a much better alternative, satisfying your hunger pains with protein as well as your savory craving; maximum one small handful	Raw, organic, unsalted nuts—protein in its original raw form, but again, keep the quantity low; one handful only
Ice cream—milk held together with buckets of sugar; most people can't digest dairy properly, lowering their immune system and ability to burn fat	Natural organic yogurt with almonds—contains a lot less sugar and the protein from the nuts helps fill you up	Fresh fruit—a small handful of berries and half an apple. These are rich in antioxidants and detox your system
French fries—high starch, very little fiber coated in trans fats (the worst fats of all)	Baked potato—much more fibrous and filling than fries or potato wedges; even better with some protein like chicken or tuna	Steamed vegetables—adding a sliver of organic butter helps release the minerals in the vegetables, as well as helping to fill you up
Salad dressing—ultra-high in bad fats and sugars; don't be fooled by low-fat versions or healthy-looking labels, these are just full of salt and fake ingredients	Extra-virgin olive oil—contains essential fatty acids; a "good" fat that helps your body burn calories	Olives—a great source of the omega 3 and 6 essential fatty acids that help kick fat out of your fat cells and into your bloodstream, where they can be burned off more easily, and with more fiber than oil

Bad	Better	Best
Muesli/granola bars—these masquerade as healthy but are full of sugar	Dried fruit and nuts—contain fruit sugars and some complete protein; not a bad snack!	Raw vegetables—broccoli, celery, carrots, cucumber, and cauliflower are jam-packed with nutrients and have very few calories
Cakes—loaded with sugar, wheat, yeast, and bad fats	Muffin from health-food shop—contains fibre and fewer bad fats	Fruit and nuts—contain fruit sugars and some complete protein
Chocolate bar—convenient, pocket-sized fat bomb	Fruit and nuts—contain fruit sugars and some complete protein	Raw cucumber with some avocado
Croissant—zero fiber and soaked in bad fats; probably the worst breakfast known to cellulite	Muffin from health-food shops—contains fiber and fewer bad fats	Raw vegetables with just a little organic hummus—loads of fiber, vitamins, and minerals
Cookies—empty calories, full of salt, sugar, and the bad fats lead to cellulite	Oatcake with nut butter—wheat free, contains some fiber, protein, and good fats	Rice cake with turkey and avocado—the perfect blend of proteins, carbs, and good fats
Pasta dish, such as lasagne—packed with bad fats and coated with calories from the cheese and cheese sauce	Steak and salad—a simple dish containing all the nutrients you need	Organic steak and Super Salad (see p. 99)—organic meat contains fewer toxins and zero hormones; choose a lean cut and serve with a brightly colored salad
Burger and fries—nutritionally very poor, the bread is often so sugary it's classified as a pastry, and sometimes there's not even real potato in the fries	Burger without the bun and salad—breadless means fewer empty carbs and more room for a fresh salad	Lean beef stir-fry with loads of vegetables—quick and delicious; feeds your muscles and burns your fat
Fried chicken—usually poor-quality meat surrounded by a layer of lard!	Barbecued chicken with salad—better-quality protein and a lot less fat; just take off the skin to avoid the toxins that cause cellulite	Skinless turkey breast with a brightly colored salad
Fish and chips—deep-fried food clogs up your heart and causes cellulite	Pan-fried fish and salad—remember, you can order your fish cooked in a pan instead of in the deep-fryer	Grilled fish and a green salad—this is the perfect meal; if you want to get rid of your cellulite, have this every night
Deep-fried sweet-and-sour Chinese food—the poorest-quality protein you can get; again, surrounded by bad fat and drowned in sugar	Beef or chicken stir-fry dish with boiled rice	Stir-fry chicken with loads of green vegetables—the perfect high-nutrient, low-calorie meal

Chapter 9
Your Easy Exercise Plan

This chapter will reveal…

▸ The 8-minute workout to do every day

▸ How improving your posture makes you slimmer

▸ Why exercise makes you look younger

Throughout the 14-day Clean & Lean Kickstart I want you to do an 8-minute workout I've devised that will target almost every part of your body. If you have time, follow my 8-minute workout with a 20-minute walk.

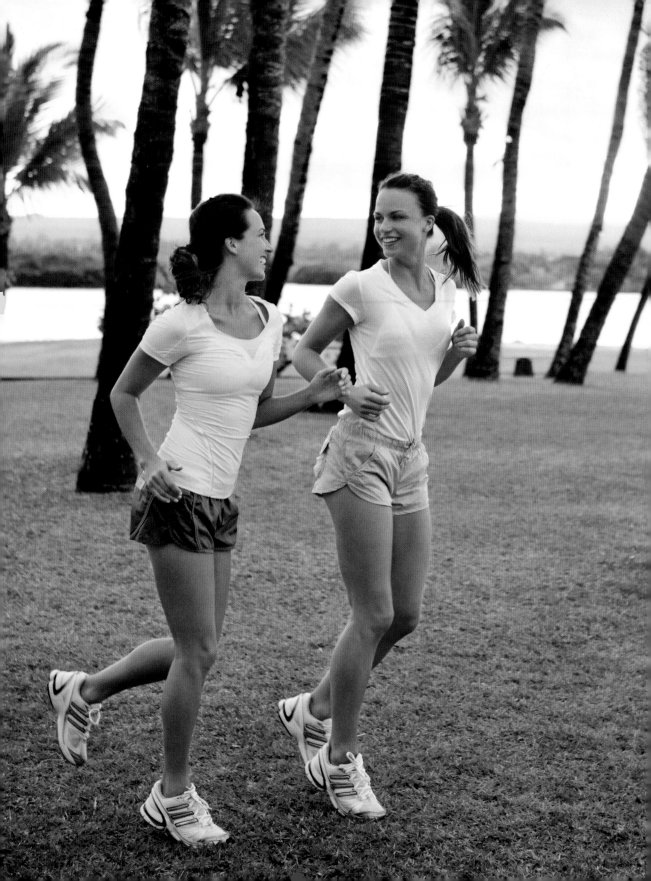

8-Minute Body Workout

A Hip Extension

This is great for your bottom and lower back…

1 Lie on your back with your knees bent and heels on the ground and your toes pointing up.
2 Lift your hips off the ground 20 times, not letting your bottom touch the ground on the way down.
3 With your hips still lifted (your body should be in a straight line off the floor), raise one knee up and lower it 10 times. Repeat the same thing with the other knee lifted.

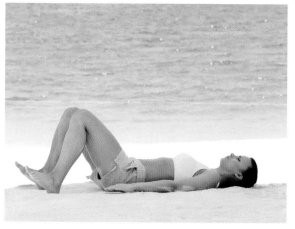

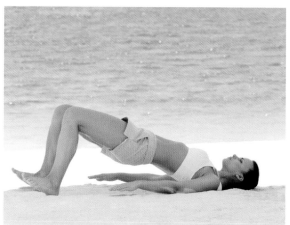

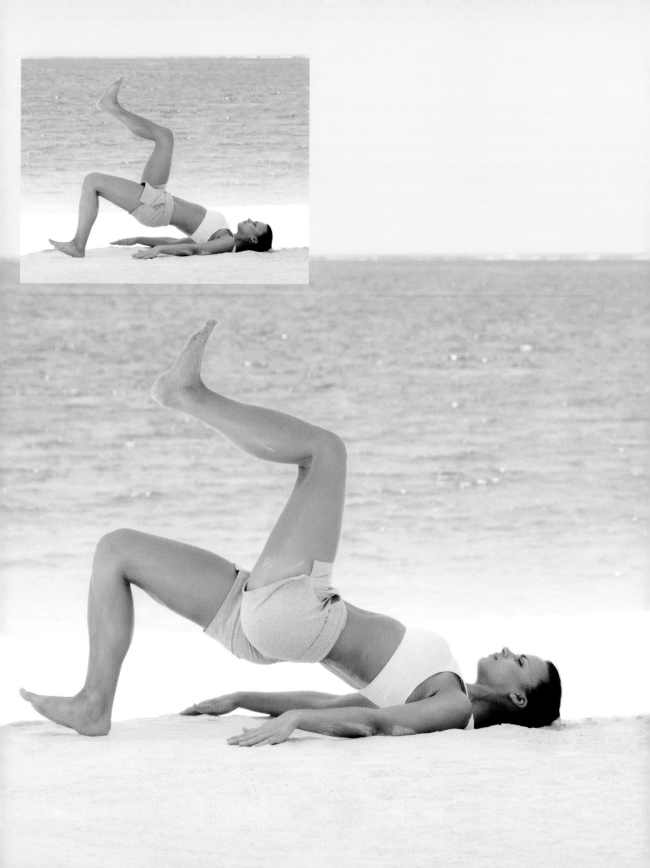

A Side Stretch

This is great for upper body mobility and loosening you up.

1 Lie on your side with your legs bent at a 90-degree angle, with your arms out straight in front of you.
2 Slowly rotate one arm up and then toward the opposite side, keeping your legs still.
3 Do this 10 times.

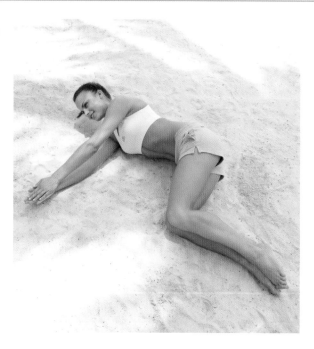

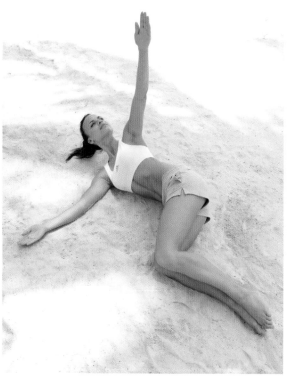

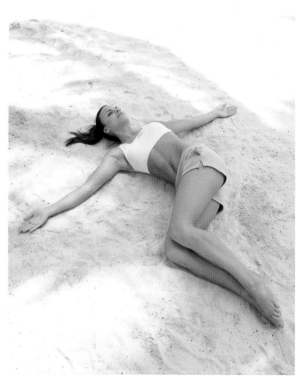

The Y&T Move

This move switches on all the postural muscles of the upper back, helping you stand straighter and longer. Good posture can take 10 pounds off someone when they stand straight.

The Y

1 Lie on your stomach with your arms up and out above your head so your whole body is making a "Y" shape.
2 Slowly draw your shoulder blades together and lift your arms off the floor. Repeat 10 times.

The T

1 Lie on your stomach with your arms extended out to the side so your whole body is making a "T" shape.
2 Slowly draw your shoulder blades together and lift your arms off the floor. Repeat 10 times.

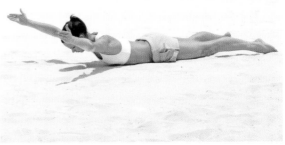

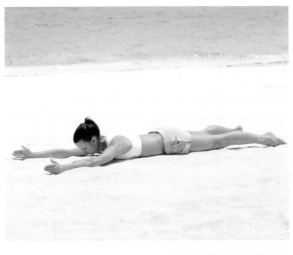

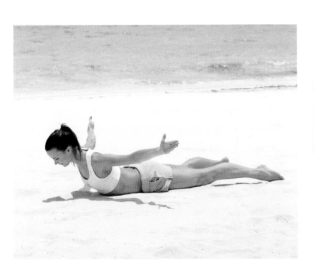

The Bodyism Tube Knee

This switches on your hip and thigh muscles and works your core (stomach) muscles. You need an exercise tube—you can buy these at most sports shops or online at www.bodyism.com. If you don't want to buy one, just do 20 squats instead of the exercises below. (See p.129 for how to do a squat).

1 Put the band around your knees.
2 Get into a squat position and bring one knee in toward the other knee 15 times.
3 Try to keep the rest of the body still.
4 Repeat with the other knee.

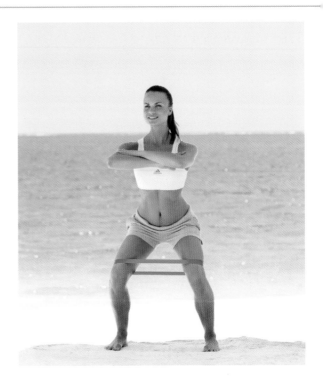

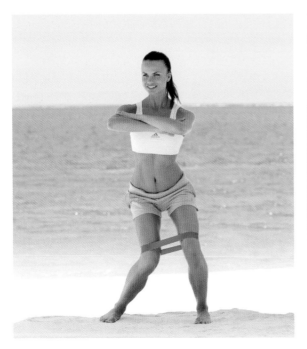

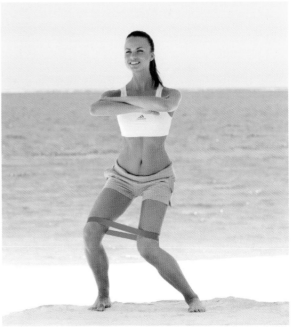

Tube Walking

This lifts your bottom like nothing else. It helps stabilize the knee, hip, and ankle joints. If you don't have a tube, just do 20 squats instead.

1 Put the band around your ankles and walk slowly for 20 steps, keeping tension in the band. At all times keep the upper body as still as possible.
2 Now place the band above the knees, get into a squat position, and walk again for 20 steps.

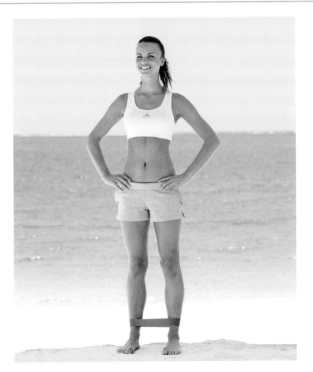

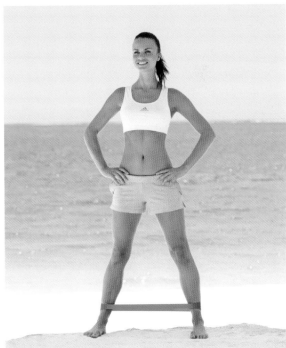

Top tip!

▶ If you can manage it during the 14-day Kickstart, do a further 30-minute workout three times a week from the list below (in addition to the 8-minute workout).

The Phases

I have four phases of exercise—one being the easiest and four being the hardest. Start with phase one and, once you can easily repeat it four times in one go, move on to the next phase.

During each phase you simply follow each move, one by one, and once you've finished, go back and start again with no break in between. Repeat a phase four times. This will take around 30 minutes. Each exercise should be performed slowly and with control. If you experience any pain, then stop immediately.

Before you complete a phase, do my 8-minute workout to warm you up. In fact, do this 8-minute workout before you do any type of exercise, including gym work, swimming, or running. It's designed to prepare your body for movement, and it gets all the right muscles switched on so your body is working at its absolute best.

Static Lunge

Great for your butt, hips, and thighs! This move uses several muscles so it burns loads of fat. And when you do it right, it will improve your posture.

How to do it

1 Stand with perfect posture with your palms facing out.
2 Both feet should face forward.
3 Contract your stomach muscles.
4 Feet should be hip-width apart.
5 Position your feet, as shown left, with straight front shin.
6 Lower your body by bending your back knee, as shown right. The back knee should just touch the floor.
7 Push up, putting weight through the heel of the front foot. Repeat on the other leg.

Top tips!

▶ Too hard? If you can't get your knee an inch off the floor, this is your goal. Work up to it safely and gradually.
▶ Don't let the knee come forward over the toe.
▶ If posture and core fail, stop the exercise until ready.

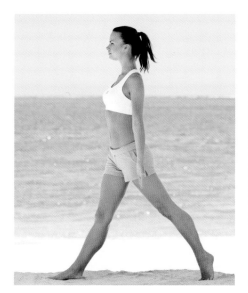
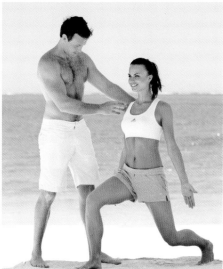

Push Up from Knees

The push up strengthens your upper body and works your abdominals, plus it's a great way to tone your arms and chest.

How to do it

1 Place your knees on the ground.
2 Set your hands one and a half shoulder widths apart and in line with your nipples, NOT your shoulders.
3 Keep your ears, shoulders and hips in alignment.
4 Contract your stomach muscles.
5 Lower yourself so your nose almost touches the ground, keeping your body straight, then lift back up to the start position.
6 Remember to keep your head up and belly button drawn in.
7 Breathe out as you push up to start position, and breathe in as you lower yourself down.

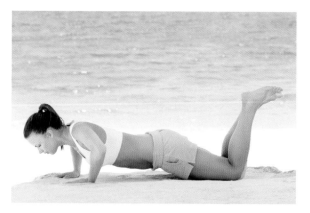

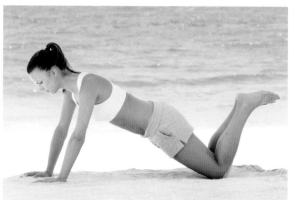

Top tips!

▶ Don't drop your head down. Your ears must stay in line with your shoulders.
▶ Keep your abs switched on and your back straight.
▶ Stop and have a short rest of around 30 seconds or until you are ready to continue, then complete the set amount of repetitions. Your goal is to complete repetitions without rest.
▶ If the backs of your arms begin to burn, stop and widen your hand position. This will place more emphasis on the chest muscles; the narrower your grip, the more the emphasis is on the back of your arms (triceps).

The Squat

This sculpts your butt, stomach, and legs, it burns lots of fat, and even improves your posture.

How to do it

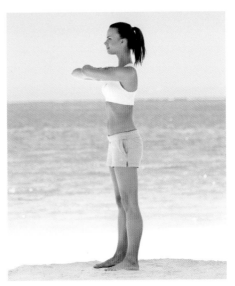

1 Contract your stomach muscles.
2 Take a comfortable stance, keeping your feet shoulder-width apart, wider if necessary.
3 Cross your arms and hold them parallel to the floor.
4 Point your toes out slightly and make sure your knees stay aligned with your second toe. DO NOT fall forwards or inwards when squatting. Keep your weight on your heel.
5 Keeping your heels on the floor, lower yourself until your thighs are parallel with the floor. Stick your butt out.
6 Go as low as you comfortably can while maintaining perfect posture (straight back, ears over shoulders).
7 Push up through your heels and return to a standing position.

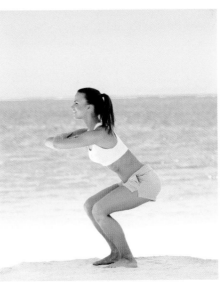

Top tips!

▸ Keep your eyes looking straight ahead or slightly above. This will help maintain good posture.
▸ Make sure you keep your bottom stuck out and your chest high.
▸ Push through your heels because this makes your butt work harder.
▸ Breathe in as you go down; breathe out as you return to a standing position.

Standing Y + T

How to do it

1 Bend your legs and stick your bottom out.
2 Keep your back and head all in a straight line, shoulders down and back, and keep the tummy tight.
3 Bring both arms alongside your ears in a straight line 15 times making a Y.
4 Everything is the same with the T, but bend down a little farther and bring your arms to the side, making a T.

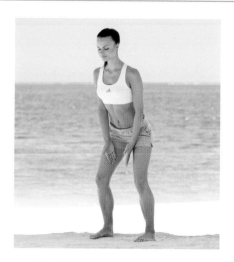

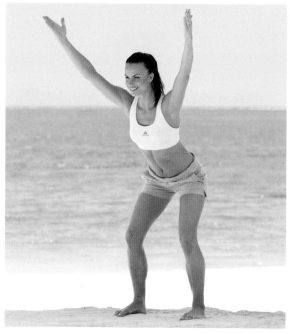

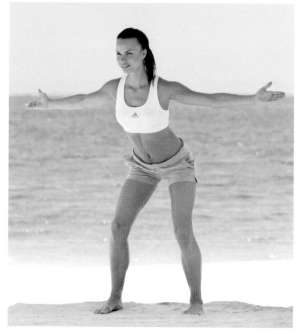

The Plank

Helping you toward a flatter stomach, the plank is also great for your back. This is a fantastic way to work your abs without the neck strain of a sit-up!

How to do it

1 Lie face down on the floor with forearms and elbows touching the floor, hips and legs on the ground.
2 Raise your hips and set the core, keeping your head aligned with your upper back and hips. Imagine a straight line from your head to your ankles.
3 Hold your body off the floor for 30–60 seconds.

Top tips!

Remember to keep breathing throughout and hold your head up.

For Phase 2, hold your body off the floor for 60–90 seconds.
For Phase 3, increase the hold to 2 minutes.

▸ Don't drop your head down. Your ears must stay in line with your shoulders.
▸ Keep your abs switched on and your back straight.
▸ Stop and have a short rest of around 30 seconds or until you are ready to continue.

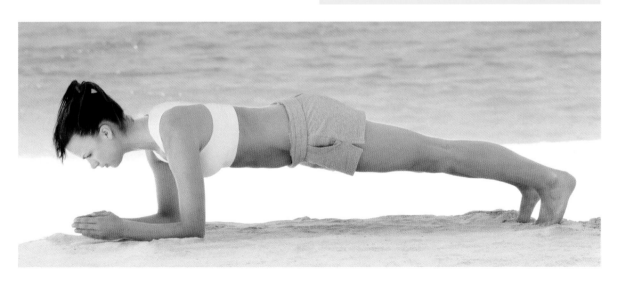

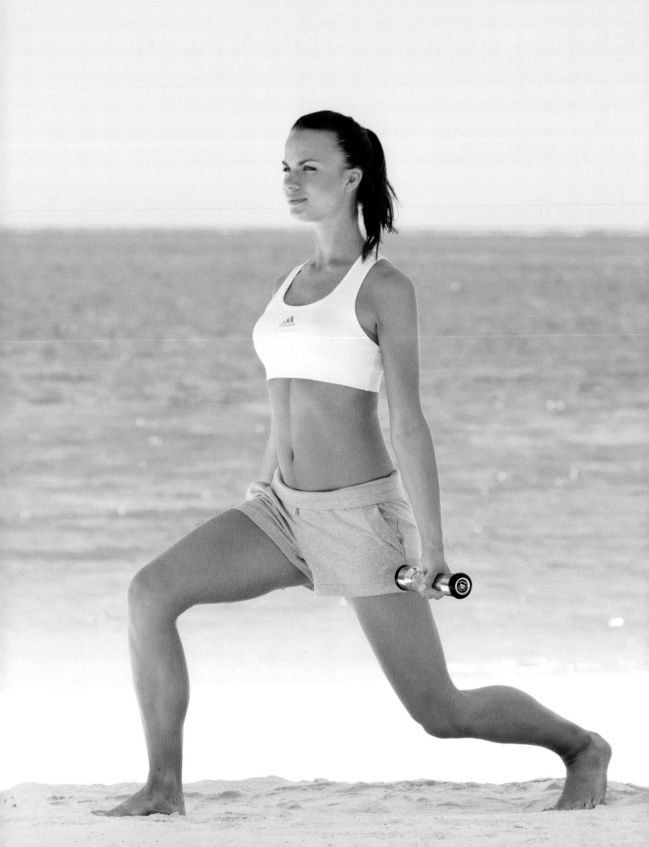

Static Lunge with Bicep Curl

The lunge is great for hitting your butt, hips, and thighs, and because you're using so many muscles you're burning lots of fat. By adding the curl, it works out your biceps too.

How to do it

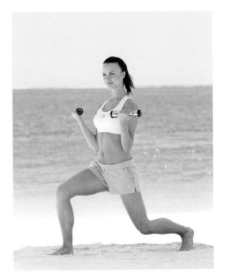

1 Stand up with perfect posture with palms facing out.
2 Both feet should face forward.
3 Set the core.
4 The feet should be hip-width apart.
5 Position your feet as shown at left, with a straight front shin.
6 Hold the weights out as shown.
7 Lower your body by bending your back knee. The back knee should just touch the floor.
8 Push up, putting your weight through the heel of the front foot.
9 As you push up back to standing position complete a bicep curl as shown, top right.

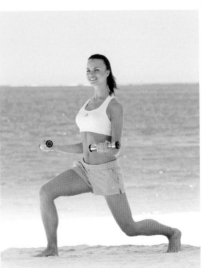

Top tips!

▸When I suggest weights, either grab some light hand weights or quart bottles of water.
▸If the front of your thighs becomes painful and tight, do a couple of extra lunges to warm up.
▸Don't let your knee come forward over the toe.

How to do it

1 Standing up straight, bend your legs slightly, and stick your bottom out.
2 Keep your back and head all in a straight line, with your shoulders down and back, and keep the tummy tucked in tightly.
3 Holding your weights in both hands, keeping your arms straight, bring both arms alongside your ears in a straight line, making a Y shape. Repeat 15 times.
4 Everything is the same with the T, but bend down a little farther and bring your arms to the side, making a T shape.

Top tips!

▶ **Don't forget your grip strength**
Lack of grip strength can hinder your workout, so keep a tennis ball or squeeze ball in the car or by the phone and work those hand muscles any chance you get.

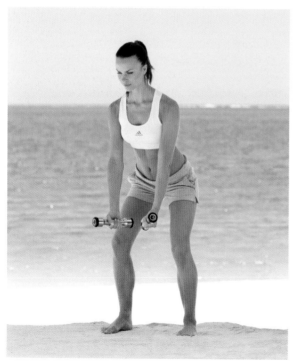

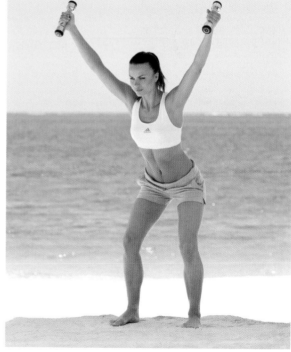

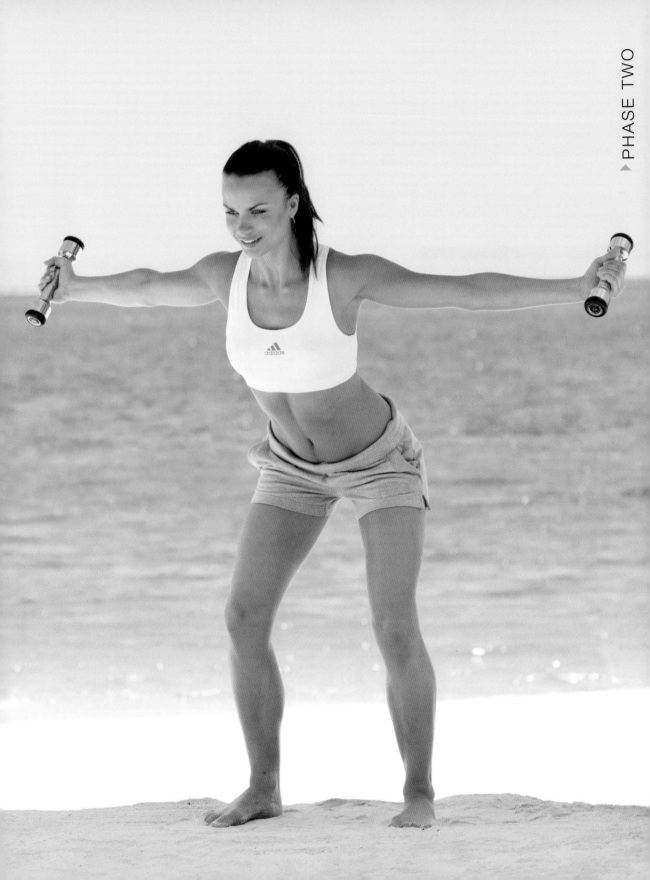

Reverse Dynamic Lunge

This is even more demanding and burns even more fat than the static lunge. It's great for your butt, hips, and thighs.

How to do it

1 Stand up with perfect posture (see Static Lunge, as before) with palms facing outward.
2 Both feet should face out.
3 Set the core.
4 Your feet should be hip-width apart.
5 Step backward as shown at bottom right. Your front shin should be straight and perpendicular to the floor.
6 Push up with the front leg, returning to a standing position.

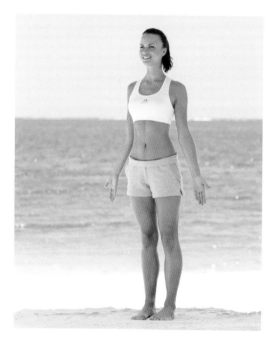
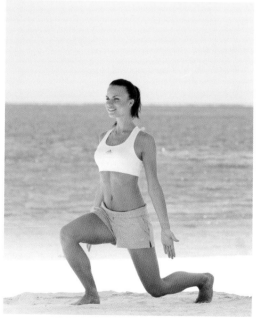

Push Up from Feet

This strengthens your upper body and works your abdominals, plus it's a great way to tone your arms and chest.

How to do it

1 Set hands one and a half shoulder widths apart and in line with your nipples, NOT your shoulders. Legs are straight with your weight distributed through the hands and toes.
2 Keep your ears, shoulders, and hips in alignment.
3 Contract your stomach muscles.
4 Lower yourself so your nose almost touches the ground, keeping your body straight, then lift back up to the start position.
5 Remember to keep your head up and belly button drawn in.
6 Breathe out as you push up to the start position, and breathe in as you lower yourself down.

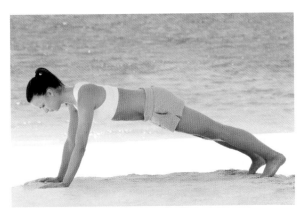

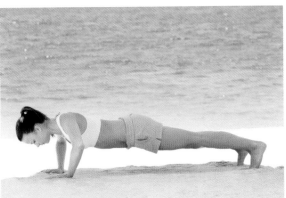

Top tips!

▸ Don't drop your head down. Your ears must stay in line with your shoulders.
▸ Keep your abs switched on and your back straight.
▸ Stop and have a short rest of around 30 seconds or until you are ready to continue, then complete the set amount of repetitions. Your goal is to complete repetitions without rest.

Push Press

This exercise works the legs, upper body, and core.

How to do it

1 Squat while holding the weight at chest height.
2 Slowly squat down so your thighs are parallel to
   the floor.
3 As you come back to standing, push your weights
   up over your head.

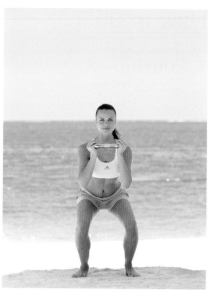

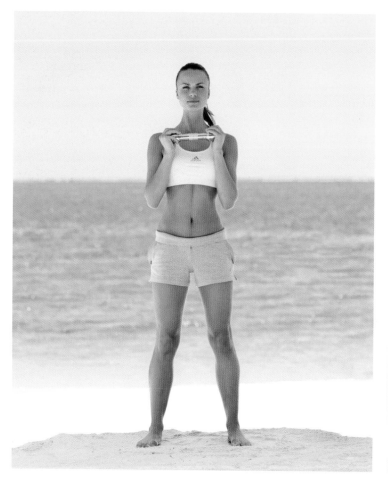

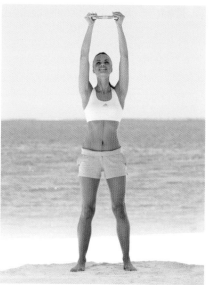

Push Ups with Elevated Feet

This strengthens your upper body and abdominals, and really works your arms and chest, too. And with your feet raised, it will work your abs even more!

How to do it

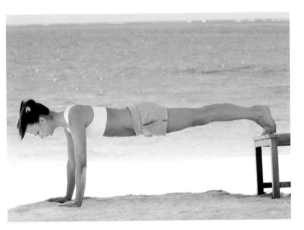

1. Set hands one and a half shoulder widths apart and in line with your nipples, NOT your shoulders. Keep your legs straight with your weight distributed through your hands and toes.
2. Have your feet raised on either a step or sofa.
3. Keep your ears, shoulders, and hips in alignment.
4. Contract your stomach muscles.
5. Lower yourself so your nose almost touches the ground, keeping your body straight, then lift back up to the start position.
6. Remember to keep your head up and belly button drawn in.
7. Breathe out as you push up to start position, and breathe in as you lower yourself down.
8. Repeat 20 times.

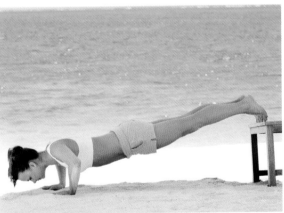

Top tips!

▶ Don't drop your head down. Your ears must stay in line with your shoulders.
▶ Keep your abs switched on and your back straight.
▶ Stop and rest for around 30 seconds or until you are ready to continue, then complete the set amount of repetitions. Your goal is to complete repetitions without rest.

Dynamic Lunge with Rotation

This burns fat and helps improve balance.

How to do it

1 Stand up with perfect posture with palms
  facing outward.
2 Both feet should face outward.
3 Set the core.
4 Your feet should be hip-width apart.
5 Step forward as shown. Your front shin should
  be straight and perpendicular to the floor.
6 Rotate your hips while maintaining core
  balance.
7 Push up with the front leg, returning to the
  standing position. Repeat using the opposite leg.

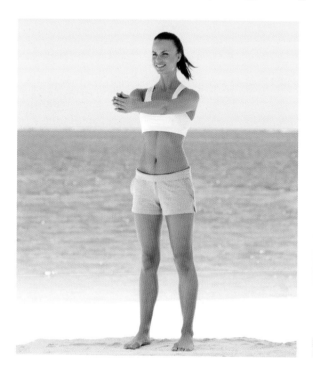
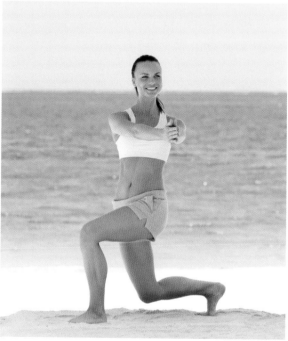

One-legged Plank

How to do it

1 Lie face down on the floor with forearms and elbows touching the floor, hips and legs on the ground.
2 Raise your hips and set the core, keeping your head aligned with your upper back and hips. Imagine a straight line from your head to your ankles.
3 Now lift one leg off the floor so the foot hovers a few inches off the floor and the hip stays level.
4 Hold your body off the floor.
5 Slowly lower your body to the floor for 10 seconds.
6 Repeat using the opposite leg.

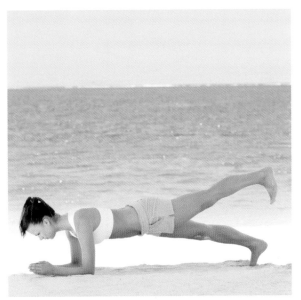

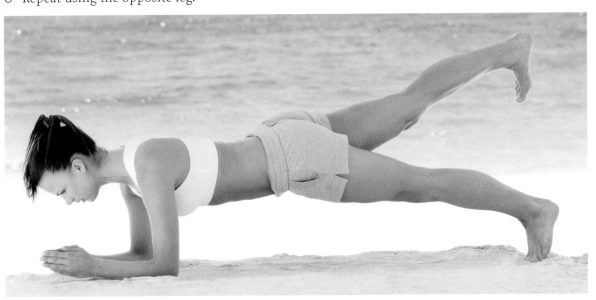

Dynamic Lunge with Shoulder Press

Adding a few extra movements burns even more fat as well as improving core balance.

How to do it

1 Stand up with perfect posture with palms facing outward.
2 Both feet should face outward.
3 Set the core.
4 Your feet should be hip-width apart.
5 Step forward as shown opposite, bending your arms at the elbows. Your front shin should be straight and perpendicular to the floor.

6 Push up with the front leg, returning to the standing position, see bottom right.
7 As you come up, straighten your arms to lift the weights back up again, see bottom left.

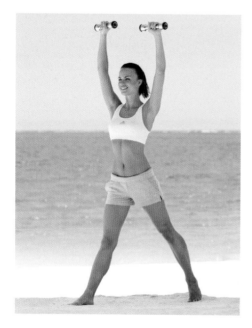

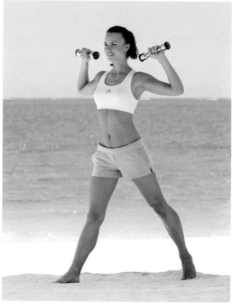

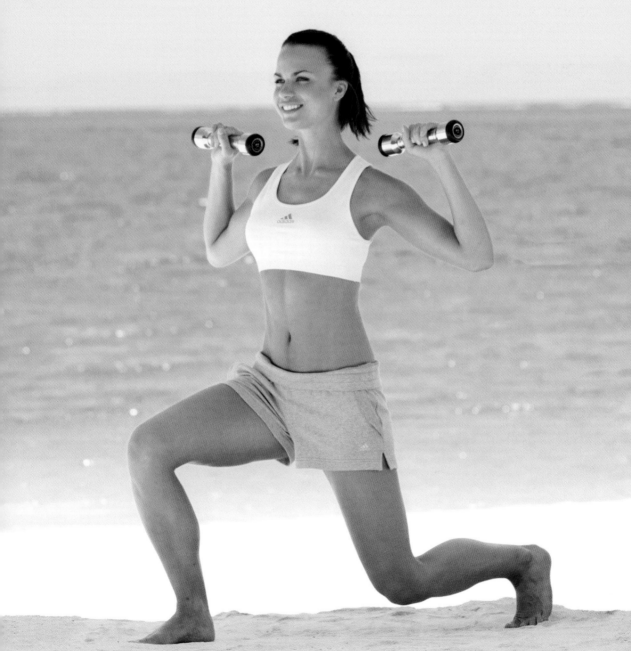

Single-legged Squat

This is an excellent all-round exercise and fantastic for posture.

How to do it

1 Set the core.
2 Take a comfortable stance, keeping your feet shoulder-width apart, or wider if necessary.
3 Join your hands and hold your arms parallel to the floor.
4 Point your toes out slightly and make sure your knees stay aligned with your second toe.
5 Lift one leg off the floor and squat down. DO NOT fall forward when squatting.
6 Don't let the leg that is working buckle inward.
7 Repeat 10 times on each leg.

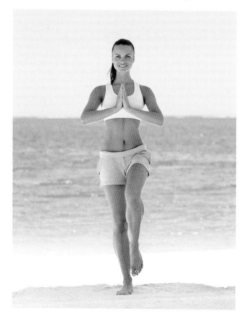 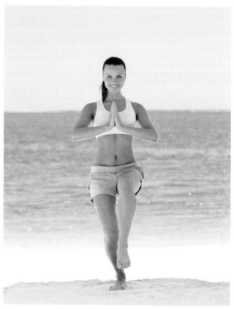

Single-legged Push Up

This strengthens your upper body and works your abdominals when done properly. It's also a great way to tone your arms and chest. By using only one leg, the body is forced to use the stomach muscles more (to keep it steady).

How to do it

1 Set your hands one and a half shoulder widths apart and in line with your nipples, NOT your shoulders.
2 Set perfect posture with your ears, shoulders, and hips in alignment.
3 Set the core.
4 Lower yourself for around 2 seconds keeping your body straight.
5 Remember to keep your head up and belly button drawn in.
6 Breath out as you push up to the start position.

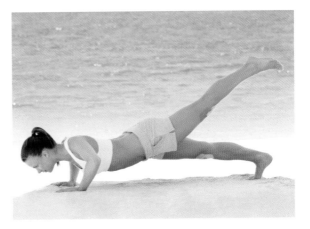

Top tips!

▶ Work up to repeating the exercise 10 times with each foot lifted, see photos at right.
▶ If the backs of your arms begin to burn, stop and widen your hand position. This will place more emphasis on the chest muscles; the narrower your grip, the more the emphasis on the back of your arms (triceps).

Burpies

This exercise is great for developing coordination between the upper and lower body. It's also a great fat burner along with really working your legs and core.

How to do it

1 Start in a push-up position with weight equally distributed between your hands and feet.
2 Jump your feet toward hands, and then stand straight up with your hands in the air and then jump—as you land, ensure that the weight is equally distributed on each foot and that your landing is soft.
3 Once you have finished the jump, place your hands on the floor beside your feet and jump your feet back into the original start position, keeping your back straight and abs tight.
4 Repeat 20 times.

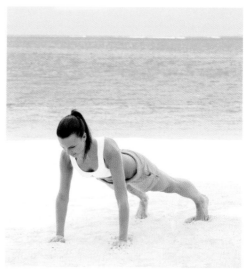

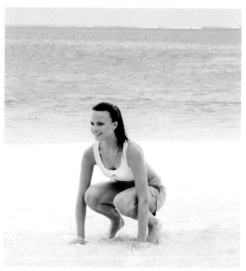

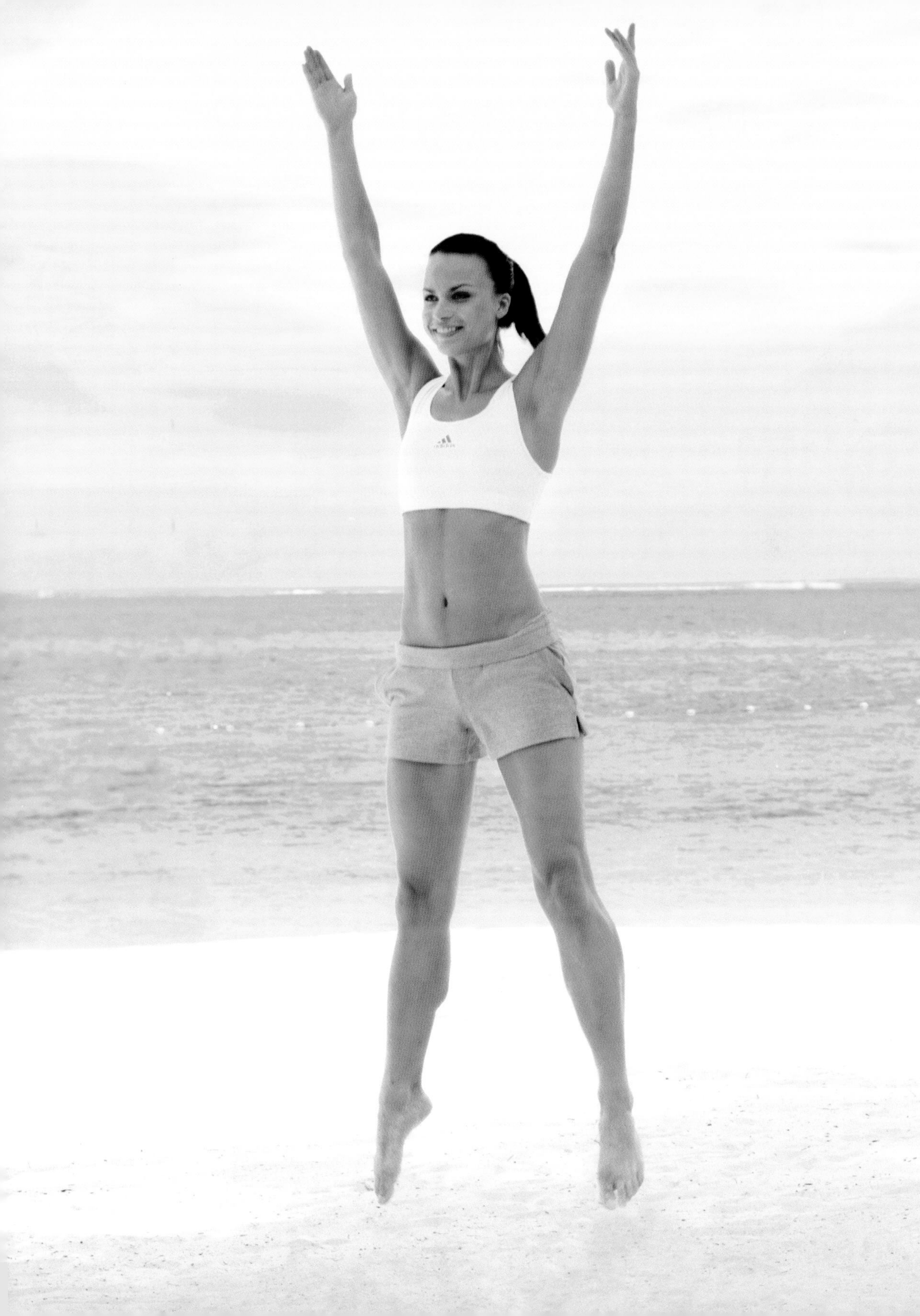

Your Post-Workout Stretches

You don't have to do these after your 8-minute workout,
but do them after every full workout.

The Skinny Stretch

1 Start off seated with the front leg bent at
90 degrees and back leg at 90 degrees.
2 Keeping your chest up, gently lean forward,
keeping a curve in your lower back.
3 You should feel a stretch in your hips
and bottom.

4 Lean back and feel a stretch through the
front of your thigh.
5 Raising your arm will increase the stretch
and lengthen the muscle.

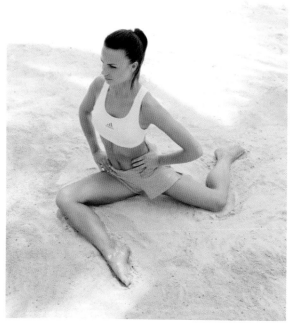
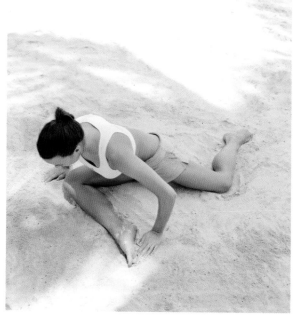

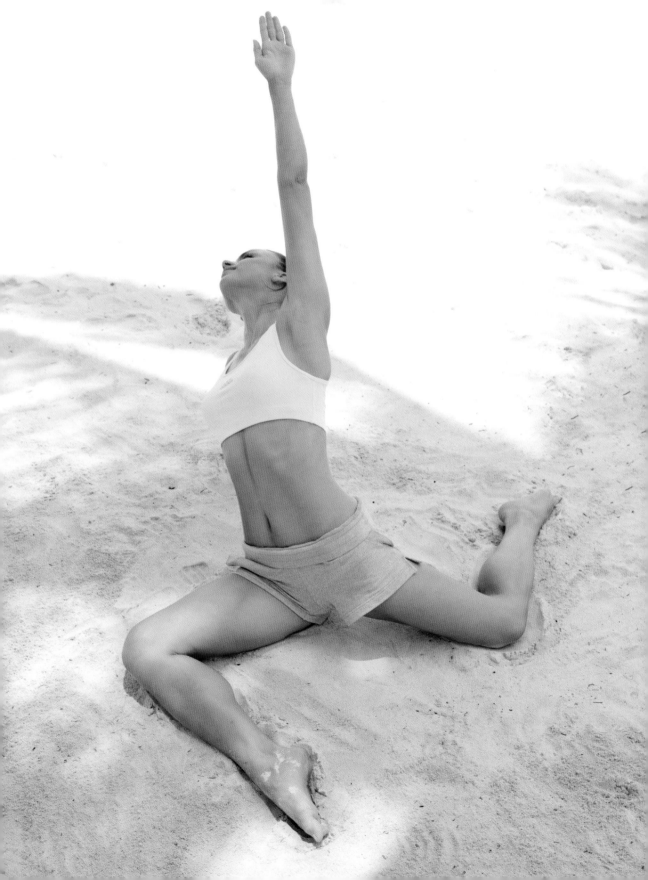

Hamstring Stretch

This stretch is great for loosening up tight hamstrings. By alternating the foot position, all the different areas of the muscle are stretched.

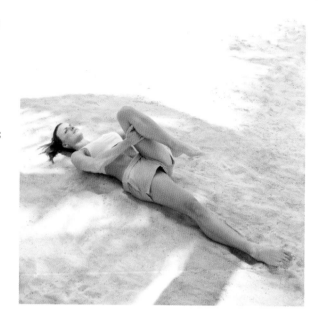

1 Start by lying on your back. Place your hands behind your bent knee, then slowly lift your leg, ensuring that it remains straight and your toes are pointing towards your head. The other leg should remain straight and in contact with the floor at all times, to ensure your hips stay flat.

2 Once you feel a stretch in the hamstring, hold for 30–60 seconds.

3 After the first sequence is complete, slowly turn the toe out and hold for 30–60 seconds. Then turn the toe in and switch legs.

4 If you feel pain in your lower back, roll a towel and place it under your lower back for support.

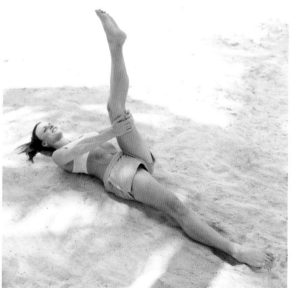

Top tip!

▶ **Breathe from your belly**
When you're exercising, keep a straight, perfect posture and focus on taking deep breaths from your belly and not your chest (your lower tummy should puff out when you breathe properly, not your chest).

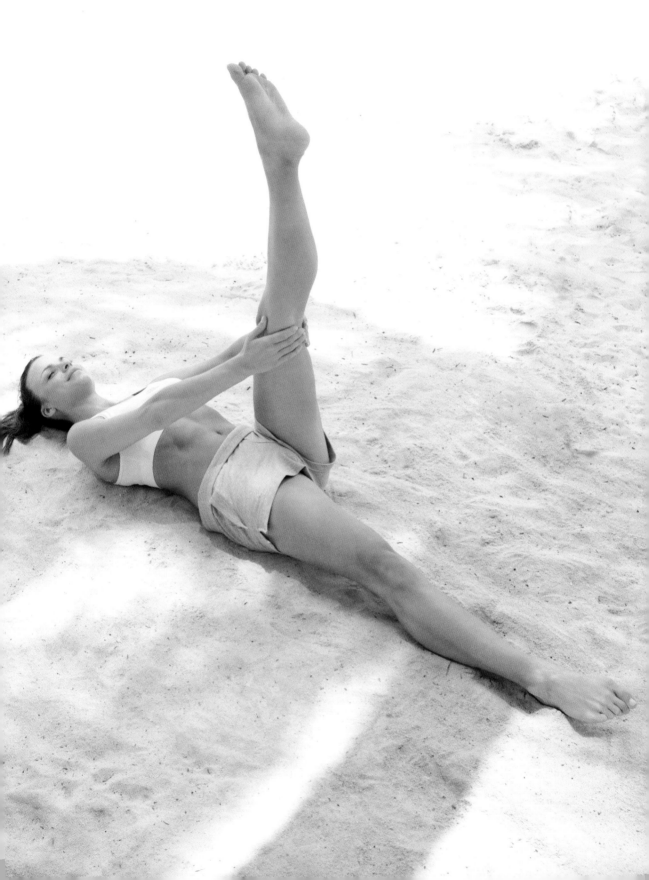

Chapter 10
Staying Clean & Lean For Life

This chapter will reveal…

▸ A reminder of the Clean & Lean basics

▸ The "cheat meal"

▸ How not to talk yourself tired

So you've got this far—well done! If you've followed my 14-day Clean & Lean Kickstart while reading the last nine chapters, you should be looking and feeling pretty amazing right now. But don't give it all up at this stage —because I want you to stay clean and lean for life, and it's easier than you'd imagine.

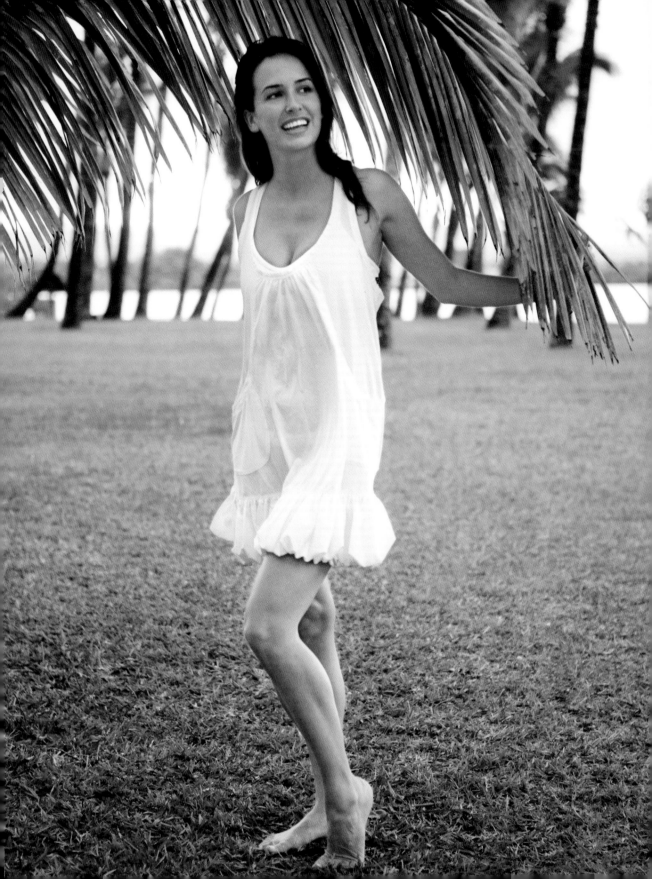

A Reminder of the Clean & Lean Basics

I don't expect you to remember—or follow—every single thing I've recommended throughout this book. And I don't expect you never to have a glass of wine or a bar of chocolate ever again. In fact, I want you to have a blowout meal once a week (this is called a "cheat meal," and I'll explain more about that below). What I do want you to do more than anything is to follow the Clean & Lean basics. Here's a brief reminder:

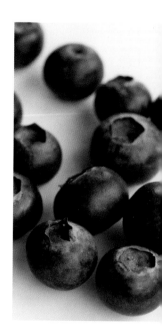

- Choose clean, lean foods and drinks as much as possible. Whether you're shopping for food, or selecting from a menu, always go for the cleanest, most natural-looking food or meal you see. If you can't recognize a food or its contents, give it a miss.
- Avoid sugar at all costs—there really are no benefits to be had from having sugar in your diet. So next time you're tempted by a pretty pink cupcake, think of the unsightly ring of fat around your waist and the wrinkles it will give you; not to mention the fact that you may well feel grumpy and tired shortly after you've eaten it. If that doesn't put you off, I don't know what will!
- Eat plenty of good fats—they will take years off your face, banish cravings, and help you to slim down your waist.
- Exercise at least three times a week—even if you just do my 8-minute plan.
- Cut back on alcohol.
- Don't stress-eat.
- When in doubt, eat fish and greens! Think, Lean and Green!
- Stress makes you fat—chill out and you'll lose weight.
- Stick to two coffees a day—maximum!

ROBERT'S STORY

"Staying in shape was never at the top of my to-do list. It sounds a little corny, but my experience of the Clean & Lean program has been life-changing. In three months I managed to lose weight and become fitter and stronger than I've ever been in my life. In fact, the last time I was at my current weight I was sixteen years old!"

Don't talk yourself tired/fat/toxic

Half the battle when it comes to keeping your body in shape is keeping your mind in shape, too. I once spent an entire year being tired without even realizing that I was causing the whole problem myself. I was working hard and training harder, and whenever anybody asked me how I was, my automatic response would be: "I'm exhausted." Pretty soon my body started believing what I was constantly telling it.

Then, one day, my best friend and I were having lunch and he asked how I was. As usual I replied, "I'm completely shattered." He just shook his head and told me I'd been giving him the same answer for a year and that it was becoming boring. This hit me like a slap in the face. I'd been talking myself into feeling tired for a whole year! From that second on, I promised myself that I wouldn't tell anyone—including myself—that I was tired or exhausted. When somebody asked me how I felt I'd say, "Amazing, thanks!" That message started filtering into my body and I really did start to feel amazing.

So don't describe yourself as tired, or fat, or unfit. You can feel amazing, you can feel energized, and you can feel slim and fit. You just have to change your attitude.

The "Cheat Meal"

I tell all my clients to have a "cheat meal" once a week, at which they can eat anything they like. (At my own weekly cheat meal I tuck into hot chocolate pudding with ice cream!) This helps to keep you on track, and it also helps you lose weight (believe it or not). This is because when you're following a good, healthy diet all the time, your metabolism stays steady. However, when you eat more than usual, your metabolism goes into shock and starts working overtime to burn off the extra food. Of course, if you eat this way all the time, your metabolism will get used to it and your body will just store—and get—fat. But if you do it just once a week, your metabolism stays sky high. Plus it keeps you on the diet bandwagon because you know where your next treat is coming from and don't feel deprived. So make sure you enjoy your cheat meal and choose the tastiest thing you can find. As I always say: "If you're going to be bad, make it good!"

And Finally

Your final Bad, Better, and Best table follows on the next page. Use it as a general guide in everyday life to help you make the cleanest, leanest choices possible (or refer back to my previous ones, for more specific issues).

Bad	Better	Best
Peanut butter	Unsalted peanut butter	Organic nut butter—e.g. almond, cashew, or macadamia
Muffin	Fruit and nuts	Super Skinny Smoothie (see p. 80)
Whole cow's milk	Skimmed milk	Organic goat's milk
Flavored yogurt	Organic flavored yogurt	Organic natural yogurt with nuts
White bread	Rye bread	Rice bread
Chips or fries	Potato wedges with guacamole	Baked potato with meat/tuna
Canned fish	Fresh fish	Wild organic fish
Sandwich	Sushi	Chicken with a salad or vegetables
Deep-fried food	Pan-fried food	Grilled, steamed, or boiled food
Microwave meal	Packaged meal heated in oven	Chicken stir-fry with five types of vegetables
Hamburger and chips	Hamburger and salad—ditch the bun	Steak and salad
Battered fried fish	Pan-fried fish with salad	Grilled fish and salad
Chicken nuggets	BBQ chicken and salad	Grilled free-range chicken and Super Salad (see p. 99)
Packaged garlic bread	Homemade garlic bread (crush some garlic on to bread and grill with olive oil)	Garlic mashed with olive oil and peppers
Packaged tortellini	Pasta with ground beef	Wheat-free pasta with Bodyism Super Ground Beef (see p. 98)
Jello	Jello with fruit	Fruit with nuts—ideally berries
Ice cream	Fruit sorbet	Platter of fruit
Jam	Dried fruit	Raw fruit
Runny honey	Set honey	Manuka honey
Crackers with packaged pâté	Crackers with freshly made deli pâté	Peppers with hummus and olives
Artificial sweetener	Brown sugar	Drop of Manuka honey and a squeeze of lemon

Bad	Better	Best
Water crackers—a thin, dead baked piece of white flour	Spelt crackers—wheat-free; usually topped with seeds, this makes a much better dipping biscuit	Oatcakes with avocado and smoked salmon—a complete meal with quality protein, good fats, and healthy carbs
All sweet cookies (most cookies on the supermarket shelf)—loaded with sugar, wheat, bad fats, yeast, with a pinch of salt; need I say more?	Crispbread with cheese—wheat-free alternative with a little protein	Oatcakes with avocado and ham—a complete meal
Pretzels—salted wheat; will leave you hungry and thirsty	Organic oven-baked potato chips—the plain ones; less salt and usually less bad fats (still not great, though)	Organic corn chips with guacamole—a wheat-free snack dipped with good fats makes a much better party snack

DAN'S STORY

"I'm a busy businessman. I travel a lot for work, and before I met James, I was really out of shape, tired all the time, and with a bit of a beer belly. On a flight to Singapore I read a magazine article about James—and Bodyism—and decided to see if he could sort me out before I turned forty. I was just over 210 pounds, which was well above my fighting weight!

James put me on the Clean & Lean diet for two weeks. After the two weeks were up, I told him that I needed to live "normally" and that alcohol had to be a part of my social life. James suggested that I give up beer (bad for my man boobs!) and stick to red wine or vodka and soda with fresh lime instead. It was reasonable enough, although it was tough giving up my beloved beer after golf and rugby.

It's been well worth it though. I've lost 20 pounds, but, even better, I've lost 8 percent of body fat so I look a lot leaner and more defined. My wife is shocked by my transformation!"

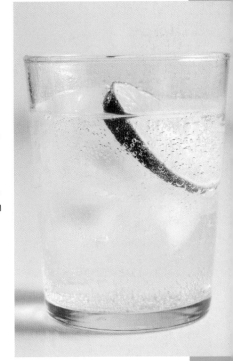

Bodyism

For more information on James Duigan's gym and
Bodyism products, visit www.bodyism.com.

Acknowledgments

All that I know and do is based on the brilliance
and generosity of some remarkable people. Mark
Verstagen and Joe Gomes of Athletes Performance,
Paul Chek, Charles Poliqiun, and John Hardy, to name
but a few. We truly do stand on the shoulders of
giants. Thank you.

On a personal note, first of all, to Christiane, for
always loving me and for her wonderful smile. And
to Elle, who changed my life so profoundly and who
has always believed in me and supported me through
thick and thin—from our first swim, when I nearly
drowned, to beach runs, Bikram, movie premieres,
and funky gym sessions, you have opened up the
world to me. Most of all, thank you for being my
friend. And to Tom, for being so incredibly good to
me—I gave you abs and you gave me your beautiful
friendship. You made it all happen and you did it
with style. To Dalton, my incredible business partner
and friend, for always being the voice of reason
and logic, and to all the team at Bodyism for their
brilliance and help with everything I do. To all our
wonderful clients, we owe you everything. Thanks to
my strange and wonderful family and especially my
sister Ruby for being my best friend. Thanks also to
big Joe Gomes for his wisdom over the years, and
thanks to the wonderful, talented, and amazingly
patient Maria, you are a special and amazing person.
Thank you Judith for always being so calm and for
taking all my calls and, last, thanks to Hugh, for
working out in your underwear and for cleaning
the gym equipment naked.

Index